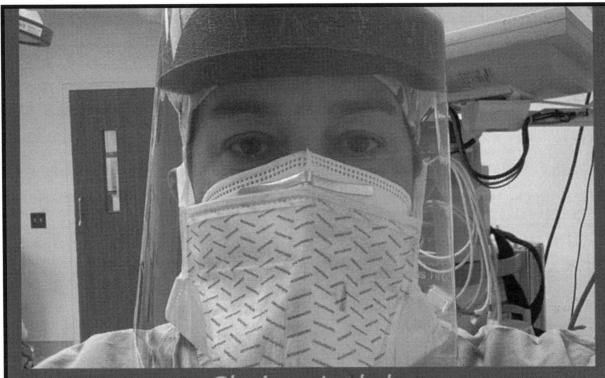

Christy Judah

Faith Over Fear

The Coronavirus Pandemic

HOPE – Faith – LOVE

Blessed is the man who trusts in the LORD, and whose hope is the LORD.

Jeremiah 17:7

And whatever you ask in prayer,

you will receive, if you have *faith.*

- Matthew 21:22

And so we know and rely on the love God has for us. God is love. Whoever lives in love lives in God,

and God in them.

- 1 John 4:16

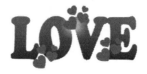

Faith Over Fear
The Coronavirus Pandemic

By Christy Judah, M. Ed.

ISBN: 9798746792228

Contact: www.christyjudah.com   christyjudah@atmc.net

Cover Photo: Leigh Sauls, RN, CRNA (Certified Registered Nurse Anesthetist. Greer, SC)

Published by Coastal Books.

Printed in the United States of America.

Dedication

This book is dedicated to my closest family and friends. The pandemic has taught us all to appreciate and value those closest to us. Among them are:

My parents, Herman (February 4, 1927) and Erika Faircloth (August 5, 1929). I will always cherish you.

My two brothers, Philip Herman Faircloth (October 23, 1958 – December 30, 2018) and James Arthur Lawrence Faircloth (August 21, 1954 -) and my sister-in-law, Rema Faircloth who is definitely just like my sister; (born March 14, 1963). I am so lucky to have Jamie and Rema during this pandemic. Living close by, we spent many hours together creating our private family circle.

My daughter, Jennifer Heather Brooke Judah Fisher, her husband, Jonathan, and my awesome grandsons: Isaih, Jacob and Elijah. I look forward to the day when they move closer to me so I can see them more often.

My nephews: James Cary Faircloth (December 10, 1979 – March 4, 2018), and Brandice Cane Faircloth (sons of James Faircloth), and Cane's wife, Brea and their daughter, Bella. I am so proud of Cane and the work he does for the coastal waterways. And Cary was such a joy to watch as he preached the gospel in churches.

My niece, Nicole Bullard, her husband, David Bullard, and children: Layla, Hayley, Little David, and Madelyn; and other relatives nearby. They are always tending to horses in need.

My dear, dear cousin (more like my sister), Brenda Sue Fisher Barber and her husband Terry of Sunset Harbor, NC, and her mom, Aunt Joyce Taylor, of Fayetteville, NC. Also her sisters Linda, Lisa; and brothers, Chuck Fisher (1949-January 23, 2018) and Donnie Taylor, and the rest of my extended family: Larry, Stephen, Karen Ann, and all the Faircloth's scattered near and wide.

This is also dedicated to fellow authors and my dear friends, Thomas and Mary Shawn Russell, a sister from another mother, of Sunset Harbor, NC. Who else could have taught me about the stock market and loved talking regularly?

I would also like to dedicate this to my additional pals and Springer enthusiasts, and artist, Jane Getty of New Jersey, and Carol Hamilton of Massachusetts; my true mentor and friend.

Even though they are across the seas, I love and remember my family overseas in Germany, cousins Drs. Mathias and Thomas Kreisler and their wives, sisters, and children. I will always remember you all. I fondly include my Uncle Wolfe and Uncle Heinz Kreisler and his wife, Tante Renate Kreisler.

Mr. Bert Lark, my lifelong friend, who died from COVID-19 was in my heart the entire time I wrote. He died alone in an assisted living facility in Vermont. Bert was my friend and taught me so much. He was 91. I miss you dear Bert.

And many others who care about me, including Jim and Annette Parsch, all my Brunswick Search and Rescue Team members from 1997 to the present, additional cousins and relatives, Toy and Robert, Bertha, Birdie, Aleta, Gen. Fontaine, Sarah, Tracy Sargent, Suzy and Tim, Shelley Wood, Tracy, and many others too numerous to name. I love you all and am so lucky to have had you in my life.

This book is also dedicated to all of the individuals, groups, and leaders who helped us get through this pandemic. The nurses and doctors literally gave their lives for patients. It is dedicated to the quiet people who set about their day to help a friend or neighbor, went to work as scheduled, cared for the sick and ill, and those who helped avoid the spread of the virus by covering their faces, wearing gloves, or by just staying home.

This disease affected us all in one way or the other. Each of you deserves special thanks for what you did during this pandemic. You were given the challenge and you met it. Some won. Some lost. Some grieved. Some just barely survived. Some sunk very low into depression or even became suicidal. Others supported them, called, wrote, or video-chatted to stay connected. Together we made it through to the other side; or will eventually. God Bless all of you who suffered in one way or another and kept on going. Our future generations care.

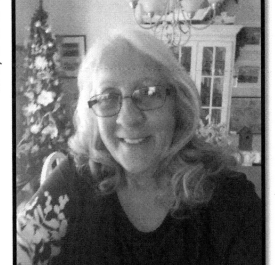

Christy Judah

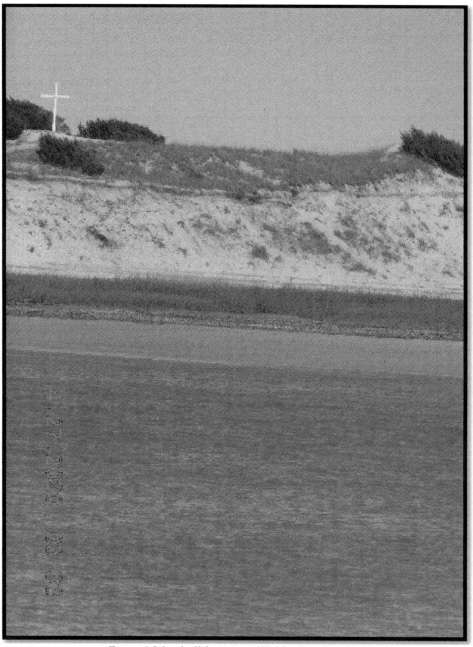

Figure 1 Island off the coast of Holden Beach, NC.

The cross on the hill of a deserted island off the coast of Holden Beach in Brunswick County, North Carolina serves to inspire and support us all. Visible from Browns Landing in Brunswick County, North Carolina, people visit to just look at the waterway for the peace it brings reminding us to put *Faith over Fear*.

Panic and Tyranny Poem[1]

By Mary Shawn Russell, Sunset Harbor, North Carolina

The invisible enemy swept across the earth.

It did not discriminate between breed, creed or birth.

Adjustments in lifestyles were made

and most individuals moved into quarantine.

In the year 2020, this Chinese disease was called COVID-19!

More than just the deadly virus was exposed across the land.

The character of the American people was evident,

so many took a stand.

Like the British forced the sale of their goods during the Revolutionary War,

we have decided not to purchase Chinese products

from here and afar!

During this unusual Presidential election year,

some cruel politicians used this virus as a tool

to cause chaos and fear!

America will continue to fight this weapon of disease,

sending hope and good health to everyone, including the Chinese!

---

[1] Panic and Tyranny Poem. By Mary Shawn Russell. Sunset Harbor, North Carolina. May 1, 2020.

Table of Contents

Romans 10:17 –

So faith comes from hearing, and hearing through the word of Christ.

Table of Figures

Be completely humble and gentle; be patient,

bearing with one another in love.

Ephesians 4:2

The Pandemic

By Annette Parsch, of Supply, North Carolina

We're all in this together,
But stay apart.
Keep the faith,
But don't go to church.
Stay at home! Wash your hands!

Buy food for two weeks,
But the shelves are empty.
Hoarding is rampant
In a "*Me First*" world.
Stay at home! Wash your hands!

Schools closed.
Businesses closed
Restaurants closed.
Life as we know it is suffocating.
Stay at home! Wash your hands!

Too many sick.
No beds.
No masks.
No gloves.
No cure.
Stay at home! Wash your hands!

The numbers keep rising.
The death toll keeps rising.
The invisible enemy
Is winning the war
And all we can do is
Stay at home! Wash our hands!

Introduction

COVID-19 Pandemic

With the global outbreak of the disease pandemic, Coronavirus-19 (COVID-19), a new world way of life was born. This pandemic infected people across the globe and spread so quickly that no one had time to develop vaccines or protocols before we found that it took over our lives and daily living practices. Coronavirus is a collection of various viruses causing illness from the common cold to more serious illness such as pneumonia, MERS (Middle East Respiratory Syndrome), and SARS (Severe Acute Respiratory Syndrome). The Coronavirus-19 was presented as a new mutation of the corona; never before known and now called COVID-19.

COVID-19 was first known to be in existence in China in December 2019. Borders of the United States were closed to certain countries to try to avoid the spread of COVID-19 in early February. By March 11, 2020 the virus was characterized as a pandemic by the World Health Organization (WHO). This was the forth pandemic in the past 100 years in the United States. The others included: Smallpox (eradicated in 1972), Yellow Fever (vaccination available if visiting countries where it still exists), Polio (vaccination available since 1955 with last known case in 1979 in the U. S.), H1N1 - Swine Flu (flu shots available but still circulating in the U. S.) and SARS-CoV-2 virus, COVID-19 (vaccines being administered in 2021.)

The Coronavirus is known in another version in the dog world and vaccinations are available for puppies and given by any reputable breeder; but this form of the virus is a mutated form of corona. The jump from canine to human was not ever suspected or known and not determined to be the source initially. This text will discuss the possible sources in later chapters. Whether the release of this virus happened through mutations involving bats or through an escape from research labs, the world would never be the exactly the same until it is under control and a vaccine is developed and widely administered. This would happen by late December 2020 and vaccinations would begin by January-March of 2021.

This book has a three-fold purpose. First, it is certainly a therapeutic way to get through the daily grind of staying put with our stay-at-home orders. Secondly, it offers the opportunity to document the infection, research, development of therapies, and healing of our state, country and world. Thirdly, this book provides a document to follow the progression of the journey of the pandemic through statistics and stories of individuals who lived through it. Most of all, this book provides a piece of history written; created as it was lived through the eyes of the author.

This book is not intended to be a scientific research into the Coronavirus. It is not intended to be a political view of who did what and who said this or that. It is certainly not intended to be a medical view or treatment recommendations for the virus. It is not intended to point fingers at any individual or country, but rather an opportunity to document what this particular writer experienced in her community as she lived through the pandemic, while hearing reports about others across the globe. It is intended to be inclusive rather than a personal account, and a way for others to share their experiences. It is with a sad and a glad heart that it is penned for future generations to remember this challenging time in history.

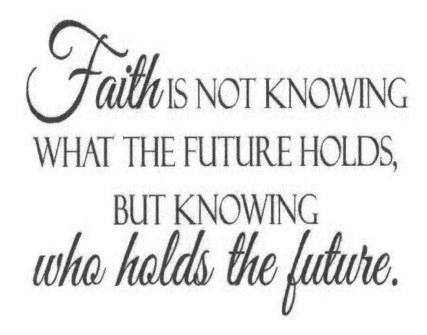

Hebrews 11:6 –

And without faith it is impossible to please him,

for whoever would draw near to God must believe that he exists

and that he rewards those who seek him.

The Corona Virus

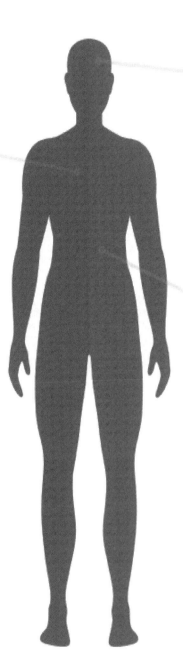

Severe Symptoms

Pneumonia

Kidney Failure

Death

Symptoms may range from mild to severe

Fever or Chills

(100.4 and up, Fahrenheit)

Cough

Shortness of Breath/ Breathing Difficulties

Body Aches and Muscle Pains

Fatigue

Headache

New loss of taste or smell

Sore throat

Congestion or runny nose

Nausea or vomiting

Diarrhea

1 Symptom Chart.

Chapter 1

Coronavirus Emerges

Background[2]

The 2019–20 coronavirus pandemic is coronavirus disease 2019 (COVID-19) caused by the severe acute respiratory syndrome coronavirus 2 (SARS-CoV-2). The disease was first identified in Wuhan, Hubei, China in December 2019.[3]

Disease: Coronavirus disease 2019 (COVID-19)

Virus strain: Severe acute respiratory syndrome coronavirus 2 (SARS-CoV-2)

First case: December 1, 2019

December 31, 2019 - Cases of pneumonia detected in Wuhan, China, was first reported to the World Health Organization (WHO). During this reported period, the virus was unknown. The cases occurred between December 12 and December 29, according to Wuhan Municipal Health Department.[4] At least this is what was publicly reported.

Origin: Wuhan, Hubei, China

Symptoms: Initial flu-like symptoms, such as fever, coughing, breathing difficulties, fatigue, and myalgia (muscle pain).

Incubation period: 1-14 days.

*Mode of transmission: Human-to-human transmission via respiratory droplets (*thought to be within six feet) or if the individual touches an infected surface or object; then, touches his/her nose, eyes or mouth.

---

[2] https://www.cdc.gov/coronavirus/2019-ncov/index.html
[3] wikipedia.org
[3] CNN Health https://www.cnn.com/2020/02/06/health/wuhan-coronavirus-timeline-fast-facts/index.html
[4] CNN Health. https://www.cnn.com/2020/02/06/health/wuhan-coronavirus-timeline-fast-facts/index.html

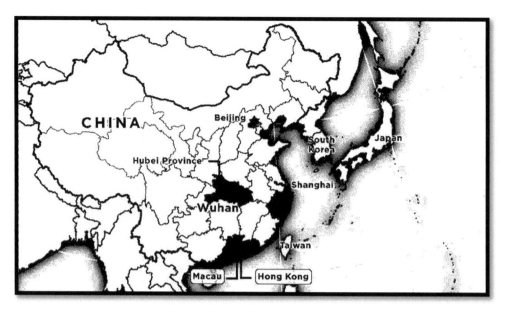

Figure 2 Map of China with Wuhan.

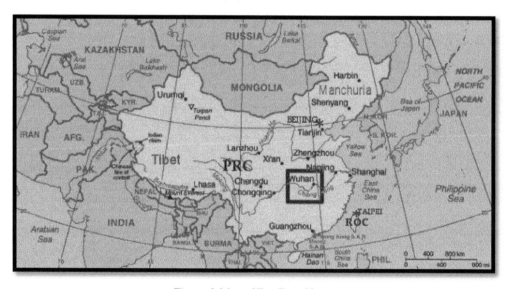

Figure 3 Map of Far East China.

January 2020[5] Huanan Seafood Wholesale Market in China

January 1, 2020 - Initially the Chinese authorities reported that this was an animal to human transmission. As a result, the Chinese health authorities closed the Huanan Seafood

---

[5] CNN Health. https://www.cnn.com/2020/02/06/health/wuhan-coronavirus-timeline-fast-facts/index.html

Wholesale Market after it is thought that wild animals sold there may be the source of the virus.

China authorities tried to say that 'the origins of the virus were the wet markets in Wuhan.' Reports to that end were debunked as of July 2020. However, those markets appear to be the epitome of unhealthy food processing and sales. The live animal and seafood markets in the Wuhan area of Huanan, also known as the Huanan Seafood Wholesale Market, has over 1000 vendors selling seafood as well as other animals including dogs and wild animals, some considered endangered. The unsanitary conditions with live and dead animals in close proximity shows animals openly slaughtered with carcasses skinned at the market. Imagine the smells with the poor ventilation and garbage piled on wet floors.

In addition to seafood, various food items were sold at the market and included:

Badgers	Bamboo rats	Beavers
Camel	Chickens	Civets
Crocodiles	Dogs	Donkeys
Emmental cheese	Foxes	Frogs
Giant salamanders	Hedgehog	Herbs
Marmots	Ostrich	Otters
Pangolins	Peacocks	Pheasants
Pigs	Porcupines	Rabbit organs
Sheep	Snakes (including Bungarus multicinctus)	
Spices	Spotted deer	Turtles
Vegetables	Wolf puppies	

Some sellers also offer unusual wares including a deer penis for £44 (about $61.00) or the penis of a crocodile for under £5 (almost $7.00).

This led to the hypothesis that bats were the source of the virus that underwent mutations from the viral strains in snakes. The virus then jumped to the humans from bats. Samples of the animals in the market and wild animals were tested and the virus was found in 33 of the 585 Chinese samples. This pretty well disputed the source as being the markets. The markets were closed for a time but reopened by April 14 2020.

Images Reveal What a Wuhan 'Wet Market' Looks Like Amid Coronavirus Outbreak[6]

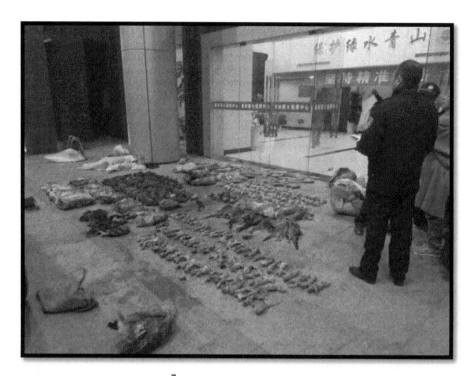

[7]   Figure 4 Wet Markets.

The images shown above were taken prior to the closure of the market by Chinese officials and show the unsanitary conditions of the live animals that were living there while the food emporium still traded.

Gao Fu, director of China Center for Disease Control and Prevention, blamed the site for the killer illness, saying: "The origin of the new coronavirus is the wildlife sold illegally in a Wuhan seafood market." He added that it was clear 'this virus is adapting and mutating'.

Many cities including Guangzhou, Shenzhen, and Beijing have banned sales of live poultry and animals in their downtown area, but the markets are still common across the country.

---

[6] Images Reveal What A Wuhan 'Wet Market' Looks Like Amid Coronavirus Outbreak. Ladbible.com.
[7] Chinese Wet Market. Barelyablog.com.

An estimated 56 million people went on lockdown in China to stop coronavirus spreading, with experts warning the virus was uncontrollable and putting pressure on already packed hospitals.

After the original case in December 2019, 41 additional people were identified with COVID by January 2, 2020. Because all were not in the markets, the markets were eliminated as the primary source of the virus.

Scientists are still unclear on the spread of the virus, which has been noted for to its similarity to SARS (Severe Acute Respiratory Syndrome), which killed nearly 650 people back in 2002-2003. Bio-warfare is one theory still being investigated. By June of 2021, the bio-warfare theory, dismissed by lead officials in 2020 is now under active discussion by some leaders who dismissed it in 2020. Even emails are being scrutinized between American officials and Chinese lab officials, namely Anthony Fauci, to gather additional data. New information is coming to light in June of 2021 about illness in the lab in Wuhan as early as November, even possibly earlier, some lab workers in the Chinese lab were ill.

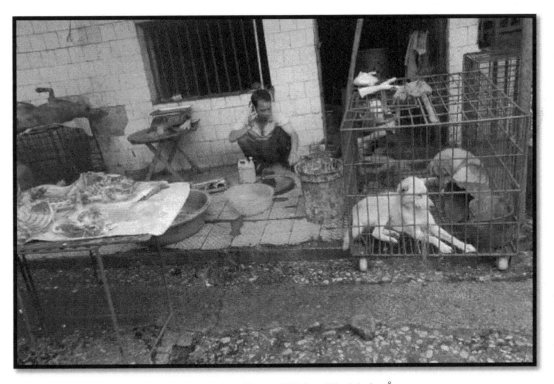

Figure 5 Wuhan Wet Market.[8]

---

[8] Business Insider.

January[9] 2020

In early January, no one could even imagine what was in store for the United States and the rest of the world. On January 5th China announced that the pneumonia cases in Wuhan were not SARS or MERS. The Wuhan Municipal Health Commission said an investigation has been started into this matter. In two days, they identified the virus as coronavirus, initially named 2019-nCoV by the World Health Organization (WHO).

The first announced death caused by the coronavirus was a 61-year-old man, exposed to the virus at the seafood market, who died on January 9th after respiratory failure caused by severe pneumonia. By January 17th, a second person had died in China. The United States responded to the outbreak by implementing screenings for symptoms at airports in San Francisco, New York and Los Angeles, initially criticized by opponents but later praised as President Donald Trump acted early and decisively in the initial stages.

By January 20th, 2020, China reported 139 new cases and one more death. On this date the first cases were reported in Japan, South Korea, and Thailand by the WHO. Throughout the heaviest casualties of the disease most believed the numbers coming out of China were under reported.

On the same day the National Institutes of Health announced that it was working on a vaccine against the coronavirus. "The NIH was in the process of taking the first steps towards the development of a vaccine," said Dr. Anthony Fauci, director of the National Institutes of Allergy and Infectious Diseases.

The next day, on January 21, the first case in the United States was confirmed in Washington State in a 35-year-old man who had returned from Wuhan, China on January 15th. The President of the United States (President Donald J. Trump) was told at that time (January 23rd) that this was nothing to worry about by his health advisors. That was about to change very soon; across the globe.

The World Health Organizations responded on January 23rd by convening an emergency meeting to discuss this new virus. It was not deemed a world emergency at that time.

The virus was beginning to spread and large-scale celebrations such as the Lunar New Year celebrations in Beijing and elsewhere across the globe were cancelled. There was a partial lockdown in Wuhan and some nearby cities in China. By the 28th of January, the Chinese President Xi Jinping met with WHO Director General Tedros Adhanom in Beijing. At the meeting, Xi and the WHO agreed to send a team of international experts, including U.S. Centers for Disease Control and Prevention staff, to China to investigate this illness. (Wuhan later re-opened on April 8th, 2020 after a 76-day lockdown.)

---

[9] CNN Health. https://www.cnn.com/2020/02/06/health/wuhan-coronavirus-timeline-fast-facts/index.html

Brian Mc Gleenon[10]

About the same time, Brian Mc Gleenon[11] wrote an article titled, "Coronavirus: Wuhan has Deadly Pathogen Lab Linked to Chinese Scientist under Investigation[12]" describing the link between certain individuals and COVID, especially a scientist working in Winnipeg, Canada. He stated that, "The scientist who worked at the National Microbiology Lab in Winnipeg made at least five trips to China between 2017-18, including one to train scientists and technicians at China's newly certified Level 4 lab, which does research with the most-deadly pathogens. Xiangguo Qiu, who was escorted out of the Winnipeg lab in July amid an investigation into what's being described by Public Health Agency of Canada as a possible "policy breach," was invited to go to the Wuhan National Bio-safety Laboratory of the Chinese Academy of Sciences twice a year for two years, for up to two weeks each time. Several of Mrs. Qiu's co-workers say there have always been questions about her trips to China, and what information and technology she was sharing with researchers there."

He continued, "One employee said: "It's not right that she's a Canadian government employee providing details of top-secret work and know-how to set up a high-containment lab for a foreign nation." According to documents obtained by CBC News during a September 2017 trip, she also met with collaborators in Beijing, the documents say, but their names have also been blacked out."

Mc Glennon said, "Qiu, her husband Keding Cheng, and her students from China, were removed on July 5 from Canada's only Level 4 lab, one equipped to work with the most serious and deadly human and animal diseases, such as Ebola. Meanwhile, there has been no change in Qiu and Cheng's status at the University of Manitoba, which had severed ties with both of them and reassigned her students in July."

He explained that "Qiu is a medical doctor and virologist who helped develop ZMapp, a treatment for the deadly Ebola virus, which killed more than 11,000 people in West Africa, between 2014 and 2016, and saw an outbreak in Congo earlier this year. She is a medical doctor originally from Tianjin in China. She came to Canada for graduate studies in 1996. She is still affiliated with the university there and has brought in many students over the years to help with her work." He continued by saying, "This news comes amid a (United States) Department of Justice announcement that the Chair of Harvard University's Chemistry and Chemical Biology Department and two Chinese nationals have been charged in connection with aiding the People's Republic of China."

---

[11] Mc Gleenon, Brian. Freelance Writer, Author, Newspaper Writer and Video Journalist; based in London, England.
[12] Coronavirus: Wuhan has deadly pathogen lab linked to Chinese scientist under investigation. Brian Mc Gleenon. January 28, 2020.

He said, "Doctor Charles Lieber, 60, Chair of the Department of Chemistry and Chemical Biology at Harvard University, was arrested this morning and charged by criminal complaint with one count of making a materially false, fictitious and fraudulent statement. Yanqing Ye, 29, a Chinese national, was also charged in an indictment today with one count each of visa fraud, making false statements, acting as an agent of a foreign government and conspiracy. He is currently in China. Zaosong Zheng, 30, a Chinese national, was arrested on December 10, 2019, at Boston's Logan International Airport and charged by criminal complaint with attempting to smuggle 21 vials of biological research to China. On January 21, 2020, Zheng was indicted on one count of smuggling goods from the United States and one count of making false, fictitious or fraudulent statements."

He went on to say that, "According to an Israeli biological warfare expert who spoke to *The Washington Times*, the deadly animal-borne coronavirus spreading globally may have originated in a laboratory in the city of Wuhan linked to China's covert biological weapons program. Radio Free Asia last week rebroadcast a Wuhan television report from 2015 showing China's most advanced virus research laboratory, known as the Wuhan Institute of Virology. The laboratory is the only declared site in China capable of working with deadly viruses. Dany Shoham, a former Israeli military intelligence officer who has studied Chinese biological warfare, said the institute is linked to Beijing's covert bio-weapons program." His startling links clearly supported the bio-warfare theories.

———

As of **May 4, 2020**, more and more sources believe that the virus was most likely accidentally released from the Wuhan Lab. Investigation is on-going by the U. S. federal investigators to determine what relevant facts will come out. This may take months or years to determine officially. While many have suspicions, the facts remain:

"In Wuhan, at least two labs study corona viruses that originate in bats — the Wuhan Institute of Virology (WIV) and the Wuhan Center for Disease Control and Prevention (WHCDC). Both are close to the seafood market. The WIV is about eight miles away. The WHCDC is right around the corner."[13] Those are facts.

"The balance of the scientific evidence supports the conclusion that the new coronavirus emerged from nature — be it the Wuhan market or somewhere else. Too many unexpected coincidences would have had to take place for it to have escaped from a lab. But the Chinese government has not been willing or able to provide information that would clarify lingering questions about any possible role played by either Wuhan lab. That's why intelligence agencies are still exploring that possibility, no matter how remote it may be.

---

[13] Was the new coronavirus accidentally released from a Wuhan lab? It's doubtful. By Meg Kelly and Sarah Cahlan. May 1, 2020.

And even then, it's unclear when or if we will ever know the origin story of this new virus that is causing death and economic turmoil around the globe."[14]

The U. S. continues to investigate the theory that the COVID-19 virus was accidentally released from a Chinese lab. Bio-warfare is still on the table. Further investigation will tell. The mystery continues. However by June of 2021, more and more information is confirmed.

White House Task Force

By January 29th, 2020 the White House announced the formation of a new task force that would monitor and contain the spread of the virus, and try to ensure Americans have accurate and up-to-date health and travel information. Many viral experts were added over the course of the next few months.

On January 30th, the United States had its first confirmed case of person-to-person transmission of the coronavirus. On the same day, the WHO determined that the outbreak constitutes a Public Health Emergency of International Concern (PHEIC).

Travel Restrictions

The Donald Trump administration announced the next day that it will deny entry to foreign nationals who have traveled in China in the last 14 days. On January 31st, this virus was declared a public health emergency in the U. S. During the next few days, travel and border restrictions were implemented. Experts from around the country representing all the major-related agencies, companies and expertise were gathered to begin to investigate, document and mitigate against this deadly virus. The infection continued to spread across the United States with concerns growing in the White House and across the globe.

The Main Players

Throughout the pandemic, various figures became forefront in keeping the public informed about the status of the virus and suggested guidelines for protecting against it. Among the initial main players were:

---

[14] IBID.

The President of the United States, Donald J. Trump

The 45th President of the United States - Donald J. Trump said, "We will make America strong again. We will make America proud again. We will make America safe again. And we will Make America Great Again!" The slogans that were heard in 2016 during the elections, continued to be heard on media as he took the helm guiding our nations defense against this virus. He spearheaded the committee and for the first several months held daily briefings on television to keep the American public up-to-date on the latest statistics, events, and challenges of the coronavirus.

While establishing the White House Task Force, he put his Vice President, Mike Pence, in charge. Pence dutifully and skillfully put together the nations' experts to tackle this national problem and determine what mitigation was needed to lessen the damages it may cause.

The White House Corona Virus Task Force

The White House Task Force, in addition to the President and Vice President, held press briefings regularly, even daily through the end of April 2020 and beyond, to keep the citizens of the U.S. up-to-date on the latest recommendations and guidelines. With much deliberation, the Task Force recommended their guidelines and adaptations to help avoid the spread.

At first there was a *14-day guideline* to stay-at-home. This was extended for 30 more days to the end of April. At that time it was extended again and it was decided that the Governors of each state would determine when to re-open their states depending upon the data outlined in the three phases of *getting America back open*. Those phases were dependent upon testing and statistical reports and were to be implemented gradually based upon data in each area.

All of the recommendations and updates were communicated primarily through television broadcasts and committee conference calls to the governors and national leaders. Most families followed daily announcements on television, anxiously awaiting the next update. These daily press conferences went on until the end of April 2020 when they were modified in their presentation to move to virtual town meetings answering questions from individuals rather than the press for a brief period of time.

Additional task force members were recruited for the White House Coronavirus Task Force in the coming days and weeks, gathering the nations brightest to manage this crisis. Among them were:

Dr. Deborah Birx, White House Coronavirus Task Force Response Coordinator; Ambassador for the United States Secretary of State.

Dr. Birx was appointed to the Task Force February 27, 2020. She had worked much of her life giving assistance with the HIV/AIDs immunology, vaccine research and global health. As the virus progressed, governors and mayors were concerned that the virus would overreach their ability to handle the patients particularly with the needed supplies and number of ventilators. On March 26, 2020, Birx sought to reassure Americans in a press conference that "there is no situation in the United States right now that warrants that kind of discussion [that ventilators or ICU hospital beds might be in limited supply] ... You can be thinking about it ... but to say that to the American people, to make the implication that when they need a hospital bed, it's not going to be there, or when they need that ventilator, it's not going to be there, we don't have evidence of that right now."

Anthony S. Fauci, M.D., NIAID Director

Dr. Fauci was the Director of the National Institute of Allergy and Infectious Diseases. He was appointed January 29, 2020. His background of a lifetime of working in immunology, infection control, and infectious diseases has made him a valued member of the White House Task Force.

Fauci has been an advisor for every U.S. President since Ronald Reagan and served in various positions in public health for over 50 years. He has been a major contributor to the research and other immune-deficiencies including HIV/AIDS, Ebola, and other communicable diseases. He became the face of the Coronavirus Task Force during the daily press conferences. He was a strong advocate for social distancing (staying six feet apart whenever possible.) On March 29th, he argued for the extension of the initial 15-day self-isolation guidelines, issued by the executive office, to at least until the end of April 2020; which was ultimately done. He was a huge advocate of masks but even local virologists acknowledged that a piece of cloth will not stop a virus. While an N95 mask might, the widespread use of cloth masks became a controversial topic which left many shaking their heads while others dutifully wore them.

The White House Coronavirus Task Force Committee Members

In addition to the Vice President, Birx, and Fauci, the following individuals served on the Task Force as of April 21, 2020. As time went by, the daily briefings became smaller in terms of media attending, with seating more limited because of social distancing. Additional White House Task Force members included:

● **Jerome Adams.** He was an anesthesiologist and vice admiral in the U. S. Public Health Service Commissioned Corps and the current Surgeon General of the United States. Appointed February 26, 2020.

- **Alex Azar, II.** United States Secretary of Health and Human Services. Attorney and previous President of the U. S. division of Eli Lilly and Company, pharmaceuticals. Appointed January 29, 2020.

- **Stephen Biegun**. United States Deputy Secretary of State. He was a businessman and Diplomat to North Korea. He was also the Vice President of International Governmental Affairs for the Ford Motor Company and on the National Security Council. Appointed January 29, 2020.

- **Robert Blair**. Assistant to the President and Senior Advisor to the Chief of Staff. He has served on the U. S. House Committee of Appropriations and the Associate Director for the National Security Programs in the Office of Management and Budget. Appointed January 29, 2020.

- **Ben Carson** . United States Secretary of Housing and Urban Development. He was the Director of Pediatric Neurosurgery at Johns Hopkins Hospital. Appointed March 1, 2020.

- **Ken Cuccinelli**. Acting United States Deputy Secretary of Homeland Security. American politician and attorney. Appointed January 29, 2020.

- **Kelvin Droegemeier.** Director of the United States Office of Science and Technology Policy. Added March 1, 2020.

- **Joe Grogan**. Assistant to the President and Director of the Domestic Policy Council. Appointed January 29, 2020.

- **Stephen Hahn**. United States Commissioner of Food and Drugs. Appointed March 1, 2020.

- **Derek Kan**. Executive Associate Director, Office of Management and Budget. Appointed January 29, 2020.

- **Larry Kudlow**. Director of the National Economic Council. Appointed February 26, 2020.

- **Steven Mnuchin**. United States Secretary of the Treasury. Worked at Goldman Sacs and Board of Directors for Sears and K-Mart. Appointed February 26, 2020

- **Robert O'Brien**. National Security Advisor. Special Presidential Envoy for Hostage Affairs. Attorney with United Nations Compensation Commission in Geneva, Switzerland, which handled claims resulting from Iraq's 1990–91 invasion and occupation of Kuwait. The amounts of compensation ranged into hundreds of millions of dollars, and were paid out from Iraq's oil revenues. Appointed January 29, 2020.

- **Matthew Pottinger**. Deputy National Security Advisor. Appointed January 29, 2020.

- **Robert R. Redfield**. Director of the Centers for Disease Control and Prevention. He has been a leader in AIDS research, practical treatment of chronic viral diseases, and other aspects of viral disease. Appointed January 29, 2020. He later came forward in an interview on television with CNN television station that in his opinion he believed that the COVID-19 virus escaped from the research laboratory in Wuhan, China. He also believes that the virus was circulating in populations as early as September of 2019.[15] More information to support this became know in June of 2021. He was the director of the CDC from 2018 until December of 2020.

- **Joel Szabat**. Deputy Secretary of Transportation for Policy in the United States Department of Transportation. Office of Aviation and International Affairs (A&I/A). Appointed January 29, 2020.

- **Seema Verma**. Administrator of the Centers for Medicare and Medicaid Services. Appointed March 2, 2020.

- **Robert Wilkie**. United States Secretary of Veterans Affairs. Colonel in the U. S. Air Force Reserve. He attended the United States War College (MS) and served in the United States Navy Reserve and Air Force. He has served with the Joint Forces Intelligence Command, Naval Special Warfare Group Two and the Office of Naval Intelligence. Appointed March 2, 2020.

The White House from Washington, DC – White House Press Briefing by the Task Force[16]

The President continued his briefings until the media became more and more antagonistic trying to ask questions which tried to set him up for argumentative answers. It was unceasing during each briefing and constantly made the President and the task force uncomfortable, feeling like targets. As a result of the constant hostility from most media representatives, the briefings stopped in late April of 2020.

Then on July 21st, 2020 a briefing was held providing an update on the status of the effects of the coronavirus in the United States. Most citizens continued to hunker down and

---

[15] CNN. https://www.cnn.com/videos/health/2021/03/26/sanjay-gupta-exclusive-robert-redfield-coronavirus-opinion-origin-sot-intv-newday-vpx.cnn. March 26, 2021.

[16] (Official White House Photo by D. Myles Cullen). Public Domain. File: White House Press Briefing (49668784683).jpg. Created: 16 March 2020.

fight the spread of the virus by wearing masks and maintaining social distancing, staying home as much as possible, washing hands often. At the same time, there was a part of the population which did not believe that masks were effective in controlling the virus spread; some maintaining that the government had no right to require individuals to wear masks reminding others that cloth will not stop a virus. This debate continued throughout the pandemic and into 2021.

Three additional agencies, presumably among many, were instrumental in the research and management of the COVID-19 battle. They are the World Health Organization, the National Institute of Health and the Centers for Disease Control.

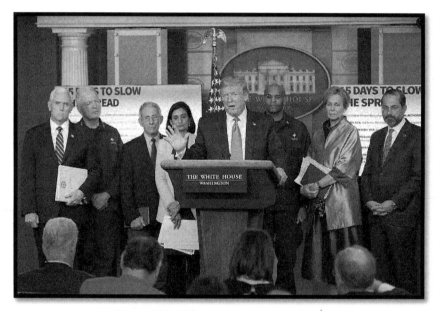

Figure 6 The White House Press Briefing.[5]

"President Donald J. Trump, joined by Vice President Mike Pence and members of the White House Coronavirus Task Force, delivered remarks at a coronavirus update briefing Monday, March 16, 2020, in the James S. Brady Press Briefing Room of the White House."[17]

The World Health Organization

The World Health Organization was formed on April 7, 1948 as a United Nations Special Agency for International Health. It is headquartered in Geneva, Switzerland and has

---

[17] IBID.

six regional offices and 150 field offices worldwide. It falls under the United Nations Economic and Social Council.

The WHO advocates for "universal healthcare, monitoring public health risks, coordinating responses to health emergencies, and promoting human health and well-being.

It provides technical assistance to countries, sets international health standards and guidelines, and collects data on global health issues through the World Health Survey. Its flagship publication, the World Health Report, provides expert assessments of global health topics and health statistics on all nations. The WHO also serves as a forum for summits and discussions on health issues."

The WHO has played a leading role in several public health achievements, most notably the eradication of smallpox, the near-eradication of polio, and the development of an Ebola vaccine. Its current priorities include communicable diseases, particularly HIV/AIDS, Ebola, malaria and tuberculosis; non-communicable diseases such as heart disease and cancer; healthy diet, nutrition, and food security; occupational health; and substance abuse.

The World Health Organization is funded by countries around the world. Founded in 1948 it acts to direct and coordinate authority on international health issues within the United Nations. Headquartered in Geneva, Switzerland, it has regional offices across the world in six major areas: Africa, Eastern Mediterranean, Europe, The Americas, Southeast Asia and the Western Pacific. The United States supported this organization and gave them $500 million dollars a year. However, after they released apparently inaccurate information on the Corona Virus, and seemingly trying to protect the origins of this virus, the President of the United States, Donald Trump, worked (mid 2020) to completely stop any funds from the U. S. to this organization while it was under review; and possibly forever. Later, on his first day of office in 2021, after defeating President Trump in the Presidential election of 2020, a new President of the United States, Joe Biden, reversed this decision. The new President and his administration will reportedly restore the United States funding of the World Health Organization.

As of May 4, 2020, the trustworthiness of the World Health Organization was in doubt in the United States, and research was initiated into their handling of the pandemic, and their apparent reluctance to assign the source of the coronavirus to China.

National Institute of Health

The Office of the Director (OD) provides scientific leadership, policy guidance, and overall operational and administrative coordination. The director of the National Institutes of Health, Dr. Francis Collins, appeared to dismiss the Wuhan lab leak theory as a "conspiracy" in April 2020. By June of 2021, his opinions seemingly evolved to include bio-warfare as a potential catalyst to the pandemic.

There are three divisions to direct and manage grants, contracts, and cooperative agreements that support research at external academic and research institutions (known as extramural research). This included the Division of AIDS (DAIDS), Division of Allergy, Immunology, and Transplantation (DAIT), and the Division of Microbiology and Infectious Diseases (DMID).

Dr. Anthony Stephen Fauci (born December 24, 1940) served as the director of the U. S. National Institute of Allergy and Infectious Diseases (NIAID) and the chief medical advisory to the president. He was also a physician with the National Institute of Health. As of June of 2021, Dr. Fauci continues to report that he believes the pandemic originated from an animal to human transmission. However, there is no proof of this.

A fourth extramural division, the Division of Extramural Activities (DEA), oversaw policy and management activities related to funding grants and contracts, managed the NIAID research training program, and conducted initial peer review for grants and contracts that address an institute-specific need or focus.

Mid 2020, grants from the National Institute of Health were being scrutinized to determine why money was given to labs out of the U. S. Treasury, to a cause like the Wuhan lab, a lab with failing inspections which identified poor security measures and less than expected level 4 handling of materials and diseases.

Centers for Disease Control and Prevention

The Centers for Disease Control and Prevention based in Atlanta, Georgia, played a major role in dealing with this disease. The Centers for Disease Control and Prevention is an agency that was formed on July 1, 1946 as the Communicable Disease Center (CDC). It began as a floor of a small building in Atlanta. Originally its mission was to prevent malaria from spreading in America.   Its budget of $10 million was a challenge to find enough trucks, sprayers and shovels to wage war on mosquitoes.

The CDC Founder Dr. Joseph Mountin pushed to include other communicable diseases in their function. It was a branch of the Public Health Service. They also provided assistance to states when requested. Disease surveillance was the primary purpose in the early years. Today, CDC is a major part of the Department of Health and Human Services recognized for its health promotion, prevention, and preparedness agency. Throughout the Pandemic of 2020 and 2021, the CDC has played an important role. Dr. Robert Redfield was the director from 2018 to December of 2020.

In January of 2021, a new director of the CDC took the helm, Rochelle P. Walensky, MD, MPH.

Rochelle P. Walensky, MD, MPH, became the "19th Director of the Centers for Disease Control and Prevention and the ninth Administrator of the Agency for Toxic Substances and Disease Registry. She is an influential scholar whose pioneering research has helped advance the national and global response to HIV/AIDS. Dr. Walensky is also a well-respected expert on the value of testing and treatment of deadly viruses."[18]

"Dr. Walensky served as Chief of the Division of Infectious Diseases at Massachusetts General Hospital from 2017-2020 and Professor of Medicine at Harvard Medical School from 2012-2020. She served on the frontline of the COVID-19 pandemic and conducted research on vaccine delivery and strategies to reach underserved communities. Dr. Walensky is recognized internationally for her work to improve HIV screening and care in South Africa and nationally recognized for motivating health policy and informing clinical trial design and evaluation in a variety of settings. She is a past Chair of the Office of AIDS Research Advisory Council at the National Institutes of Health, Chair-elect of the HIV Medical Association, and previously served as an advisor to both the World Health Organization and the Joint United Nations Programme on HIV/AIDS. Originally from Maryland, Dr. Walensky received her Bachelor of Arts from Washington University in St. Louis, her Doctor of Medicine from the Johns Hopkins School of Medicine, and her Masters' Degree in Public Health from the Harvard School of Public Health."[19]

CDC Overview and Advice

The CDC officials said, "The Corona viruses are a large family of viruses that are common in people and many different species of animals, including camels, cattle, cats, and bats. Rarely, animal corona viruses that can infect people and then spread between people such as with MERS-CoV, SARS-CoV, and now this new virus (named SARS-CoV-2)."

They went on to describe the virus as, "The SARS-CoV-2 virus is a betacoronavirus, like MERS-CoV and SARS-CoV. All three of these viruses have their origins in bats. The sequences from U.S. patients are similar to the one that China initially posted, suggesting a likely single, recent emergence of this virus from an animal reservoir." This viewpoint came into question when further investigation was done later in the year as has already been noted.

Mid 2020, the CDC went on to say, "The complete clinical picture with regard to COVID-19 is not fully known. Reported illnesses have ranged from very mild (including some with no reported symptoms) to severe, including illness resulting in death. While information so far suggests that majority of COVID-19 illnesses are mild, an early (report) out of China found serious illness in 16% of cases. A CDC Morbidity & Mortality Weekly Report that looked at severity of disease among COVID-19 patients in the United States by age group found that 80% of deaths were among adults 65 years and older with the highest

---

[18]Walensky, Rochelle. https://www.cdc.gov/about/leadership/director.htm
[19] IBID.

percentage of severe outcomes occurring in people 85 years and older. People with serious underlying medical conditions — like heart conditions, chronic lung disease, and diabetes — also seemed to be at higher risk of developing serious COVID-19 illness."

The CDC officials recommended in early 2020 that all people should be wearing masks and continued to recommend the use of a cloth face covering to keep people who are infected but do not have symptoms from spreading COVID-19 to others in *March 2021*. The cloth face cover was meant to protect other people in case you are infected. This continued to be a controversial recommendation with those in opposition of masks questioning why a healthy person with low risk of illness needs to wear a face covering. However, most follow the recommendations hoping to escape the illness.

The cloth face coverings recommended were not surgical masks or N-95 respirators. Medical face masks were considered critical supplies that were recommended to be reserved for healthcare workers and other first responders (as per the CDC.) In the first half of 2020, supplies were extremely short and did not meet the demand in hospitals or health centers. President Trump urged the private sector companies to produce the needed items and suspend production of other items not currently needed during this crisis. They did so and even companies not usually producing medical supplies began producing needed items like masks, gowns, ventilators, and other items at the same time that some companies began the much needed work to create a vaccine for the general population.

By the end of April in 2021, Dr. Anthony Fauci, announced that it is pretty obvious that the risk is very low outdoors, so the guidelines may be changed soon; especially for those who have been fully vaccinated. However, more than 5 million Americans have skipped their second dose of the vaccine and those Americans are not as protected, as they may think. Herd immunity will require that more people get their vaccines.

Ventilators, Ventilators, Ventilators

These expensive machines seem to be in short supply at the beginning of this pandemic. They are still needed by many countries. It seemed America has provided enough ventilators for everyone who needs to have access to one. Media reports were varied but the general situation as understood by this author was that once a person is admitted to the hospital and put on a ventilator to assist breathing, hope began to fade for a positive outcome of that patient.

The ventilators helped to buy time hoping the patient will recover. These life and death struggles may only be a bridge from life to death. They would not cure the illness but they did provide support for each patient while waiting for other therapies to help the body overcome the disease.

As of April the 18th, 2020, it appeared from media reports and Presidential Corona Virus Task Debriefings, that every patient who needed a ventilator had one. Additional ventilators which were still being produced would be provided for any state needing them to stockpile or other countries still approaching their peak of illness.

Social Distancing

The CDC recommended social distancing, meaning to keep people six feet apart from each other. Labels were hung, stuck to the floors, and promoted in any business which was still open to encourage customers to stay six feet apart. Later plexi-glass barriers were hung in front of cashiers and other places inside businesses to add protection to workers and shoppers. The cloth face cover was not a substitute for social distancing but meant to be in addition to the social distancing and hand washing. Oh, those dang masks.

The Spread

Global efforts by April 2020 were focused on lessening the spread and impact of this virus. The federal government and the CDC worked closely with state, local, tribal, and territorial partners, as well as public health partners, to respond to the public health threat. The CDC described the situation as posing a serious public health risk. COVID-19 caused mild to severe illness while the most severe illness occurred in adults 65 years and older.

Different parts of the country saw different levels of COVID-19 activity. The United States nationally was in the acceleration phase of the pandemic in *April of 2020.* The duration and severity of each pandemic phase varied depending on the characteristics of the virus and the public health response in that location across the nation.

The CDC, along with state and local public health laboratories, expanded testing for the virus in all 50 states which had now spread into all states by April of 2020. It was reported that cases come from travelers who brought it to the U. S. from abroad. Cases also came from close contacts of known cases and community-acquired cases where the source of the infection was known. Every state had the community-acquired type by that time. There was talk that when "herd immunity" occurred, things might settle down and get back to normal. Some foreign countries tried this approach (just let folks go about their normal routine no masks, etc.) which was later determined not to work to contain the virus. However, in late March the numbers of virus cases were declining. Then, reports of an increase in cases were noted, primarily blamed on Spring Break (when typically thousands of college students converge on beaches for relaxation activities) with many traveling together and congregating in larger numbers. The same thing happened right after Christmas 2020 and Spring Break of 2021.

With government mandated business closings, except for essential businesses (like food stores and large box stores like Walmart, Lowes, Home Depot, etc.) over 6.6 million U. S. workers filed for unemployment benefits according to the Department of Labor on April 2, 2020. This represented the highest number of claims in history. Globally, COVID cases surpassed 1 million according to Johns Hopkins University.

Initially, U. S. officials hoped to have the economy and communities back open by Easter 2020 so folks could attend church in observance of the religious holiday. It was not to happen. Before we knew it, Easter of 2021 was upon us. And by June of 2021, with stimulus checks and supplements to unemployment checks in the U. S. unemployment rates rose but business actually had to close down because of a lack of workers to work. They could make more drawing unemployment checks than work for minimal wages at fast foods and other local businesses. Nearly every business had signs in the windows advertising WORKERS WANTED. HELP NEEDED. Apply within. $11 to $15 per hour. SIGN on bonuses.

February 2020[20]

February brought more reports of concerns with COVID. On the 2nd of February, a man in the Philippines dies from the coronavirus -- the first time a death has been reported outside mainland China since the outbreak began. News reports were erupting from every direction, television, newspaper, online, and talk show voicing every opinion angle possible. Some claimed bio-warfare; others accidental escape from a lab, some animal transmission, others angry and concerned about double agents giving secrets to the enemy, whomever it was on any given day. No one really understood what was happening and most were totally confused and afraid of what the future might hold.

People were starting to wear masks, unavailable at most locations, and used bandanas or simple clothe coverings which just felt strange as this had never been needed in the past. We remember seeing Asians wearing masks for years in news reports, helping to avoid spreading the flu, and now we began to understand why they did; but still not understanding the full scope of what was to come in the next year.

Deaths in 2020

New sources at CNN Health reported the following developments regarding the China connection of the virus, fueling the acceptance that China was the source of the spread.

Dr. Li Wenliang from Wuhan tried to warn the world in December that the virus was of major concern. He ended up dying from the virus the first week of February after much harassment from the Chinese police. Many of his countrymen felt the government owed him an apology and demanded freedom of speech on Weibo, the twitter-like platform in China.

---

[20] CNN Health. https://www.cnn.com/2020/02/06/health/wuhan-coronavirus-timeline-fast-facts/index.html

By February 6th, a 60 year old U. S. citizen died in Wuhan; the first confirmed foreign death in Beijing.

On February 10th, Xi Jinping, the General Secretary of the Chinese Communist Party and paramount leader of China, "inspects efforts to contain the coronavirus in Beijing, the first time he had appeared on the front lines of the fight against the outbreak," concurrently with a team from the World health Organization, to try to contain the virus. Just a few days later, several of the Communist Party leaders were replaced in the Shandong Province. Apparently politics were at play.

On February 14th, a Chinese tourist testing positive for corona virus died in France becoming Europe's first casualty. On the same day a case was marked in Egypt, Africa's first case.

February 15, 2020 - The official Communist Party Journal, Qiushi, published the transcript of a speech made on February 3 by Xi in which he "issued requirements for the prevention and control of the new coronavirus" on January 7, revealing Xi knew about and was directing the response to the virus almost two weeks before he commented on it publicly."

February 18, 2020 - Xi says in a phone call with British Prime Minister Boris Johnson that China's *"measures to prevent and control the epidemic are achieving visible progress,"* according to state news Xinhua.

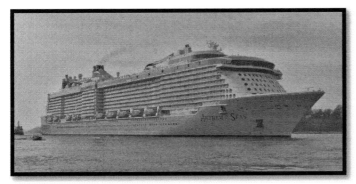

Cruise Ships

Despite the reports of *achieving visible progress*, this was actually just the beginning of the challenges which lay ahead for the world in 2020. In early *February* there were accusations by China's Foreign Ministry accusing the United States of excessive fears by the implementation of the travel restrictions. About the same time, the Japanese Health Ministry announced that a cruise ship, *The Diamond Princess* had ten guests with COVID. It was carrying more than 3,700 people and was placed under quarantine until February 19th.

On February 10th, The *Anthem of the Seas*, a Royal Caribbean cruise ship, (shown above) set sail from Bayonne, New Jersey, after a coronavirus scare kept it docked and its passengers waited for days to sail. This was just the first of outbreaks on cruise ships.

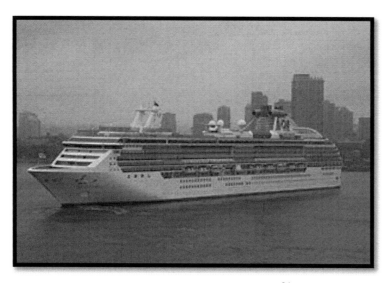

Figure 7 Coral Princess Cruise Ship.[21]

Later in April, the *Diamond Princess* cruise ship experienced an outbreak of coronavirus. The British cruise ship the *Diamond Princess* was in Japanese waters, and the Japanese administration was asked to manage its quarantine, with the passengers having not yet entering Japan. On the *Diamond Princess*, more than 700 people became infected and a dozen died. The incidents were classified as "an international conveyance.

The cruise ship *Coral Princess* had positive tested cases since early April 2020 and was docked in Miami. *Coral Princess's* numbers are currently not counted in any national figures. Other ships which had Covid cases on board in 2020 included: *World Dream, Westerdam, Grand Princess (122 infected and 7 died), Sara Costa Magica Braemar, Costa Luminosa, Carnival Valor, Silver Explorer Silver Shadow, Norwegian Bliss, Norwegian Breakaway, Celebrity Solstice, Ruby Princess (853 infected 28 died), MSC Bellissima, Ovation of the Seas, Voyager of the Seas, Costa Victoria, Marella Explorer2, Artania, Carnival Freedom* and others.

Over 40 cruise ships had confirmed cases of coronavirus on board. Many then cancelled all cruises till after June of 2020. This later extended until mid 2021. They slowly began opening back up in 2021, and most in 2021 required documentation of immunization prior to boarding. Can they legally require immunization records? Is this a HIPPA[22] violation? Oh, my. Oh, me. What next?

---

[21] https://en.wikipedia.org/wiki/Coral_Princess#COVID-19_pandemic
[22] HIPPA. Health Insurance Portability and Accountability Act of 1996 (HIPAA)
The Health Insurance Portability and Accountability Act of 1996 (HIPAA) is a federal law that required the creation of national standards to protect sensitive patient health information from being disclosed without the patient's consent or knowledge. The US Department of Health and Human Services (HHS) issued the HIPAA

First Responder Emergency Deployment
by Trace Sargent

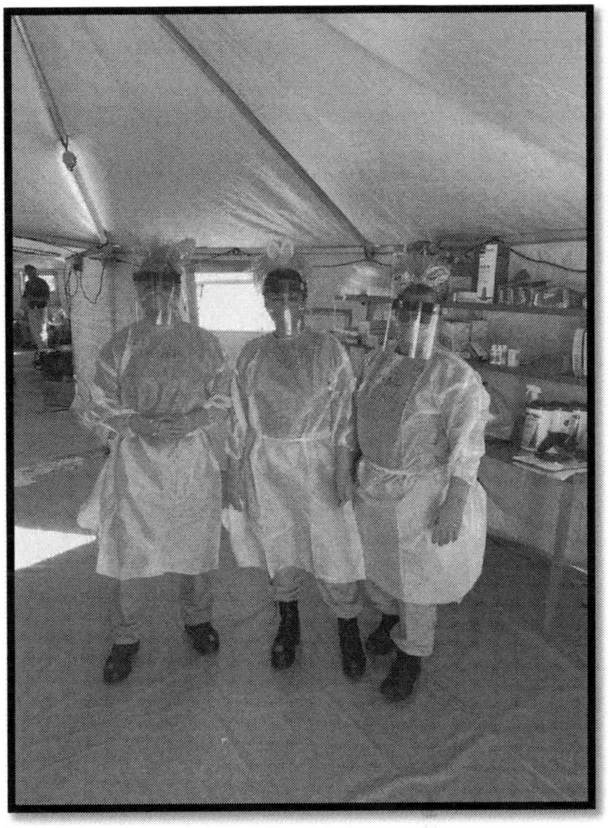

Figure 8 The Temp Team: Candice Downs, Tracy Sargent, and Lori Bell.

My name is Tracy "Trace" Sargent. I had first-hand experience as a responder with the COVID pandemic almost from the beginning of this historic event.

It was March 14, 2020. I was doing an interview and search scene with my dogs for a national crime show in Atlanta, Georgia. The story was about an Iraqi war veteran who disappeared without a trace. My search dogs alerted to a concrete pad at the house where he was last seen. And when officials excavated the concrete, they found the veteran's remains. He had been buried under the concrete for 3.5 years.

While we were filming this story, I received an email from my commander of a Federal Task Force Team. I have been a member of this task force for many years. This team is known as DMORT-IV. Although we are typically called for mass fatalities, such as the 911 terrorist attacks, we were activated to support Federal medical task force teams who were providing support and care for possible COVID patients.

Team members were deployed across the nation. I was specifically deployed the following day, March 15, 2020, to Miramar, California. At this famous military base, cruise ship passengers had been quarantined for about a week when I arrived.

Privacy Rule to implement the requirements of HIPAA. The HIPAA Security Rule protects a subset of information covered by the Privacy Rule. https://www.cdc.gov/phlp/publications/topic/hipaa.html

After an orientation and completing the required FIT tests and paperwork, I was assigned as part of a "temp team." The temp team included two other DMORT IV members and me. Their names were Candice Downs and Lori Bell. This was the first time the three of us had worked together. We immediately clicked and performed our tasks seamlessly.

We checked passenger temperatures 2-3 times a day. We actually referred to the passengers as "guests" and we treated them as such. During these temperature checks, we wore PPE (Person Protective Equipment) that included gowns, double gloves, face shields and masks. Fortunately, the weather was pleasant and wearing such additional gear and clothing was comfortable for us.

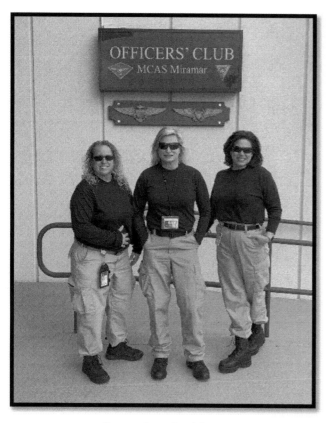

Figure 9 Lori Bell, Tracy Sargent, and Candice Downs.

Each person/family had been assigned their own room, complete with a small living room, bedroom and bath. The rooms were equipped with basic furniture and a television. Although they had creature comforts, they had been "quarantined" for weeks. As you can imagine this kind of situation would affect even the most positive person. Their morale was starting to be affected by such isolation in a strange place, away from their home and family.

Although covered in PPE, that didn't stop us from getting creative. Each day we would write words of encouragement or comical sayings across our gowns and face shields. We would also wear "costumes" that included bunny ears, bells, flowers, streamers, etc. Essentially, doing whatever we could to bring a smile to their face, and uplift their spirits.

Of course, our unorthodox approach was surprising at first to many. However, we were quickly the talk of the compound with our outfits and human billboard antics. In fact, the guests told us that our daily visits were the highlight of their days. They looked forward to seeing what we looked like and what messages we had written across our PPE.

If any of the guests were running a fever, medical personnel would conduct further testing. Their every need was catered to. They were brought food, water, personal care items, etc. to their rooms. They were allowed to walk around the courtyard of the facility, but must wear masks at all times. The only time they did not have to wear masks was when they were in their rooms.

During our two-week deployment, we met folks who lived in the four corners of the United States. They ranged from Hawaii to New York. We formed great friendships and become close to many of the guests. Many of them wanted pictures of us together and with them so they could tell their family and friends about their California *temp* team.

Although the overall experience was positive and upbeat, we did see the darker side of the COVID pandemic. An older couple who had been together most of their lives, were separated during their quarantine. Unfortunately, the husband had a high temperature and after further testing he was positive for the virus. He was medically transported to a hospital about two hours away because all of the local hospitals were full.

During our daily visits, we recognized the wife was by herself. She was a sweet, sensitive and dear woman. We always asked how she was doing and if there was anything, we could do for her. She always politely said no. It was apparent to us that she was not used to being alone, and we surmised that her husband was her rock.

On this day, we started our shift like any other day. However, the medical team advised us that the husband took a turn for the worse and was not expected to survive. They stated they were making arrangements to transport her to the hospital to be with her husband, during what could be the last days of his life and their last days as a couple.

As we checked temps down the long hallway we came to her room. Her door was already open.   I'll never forget the vision in front of us. A couple of luggage bags were sitting next to her with her jacket and purse sitting on top of them. She was sitting on the bed, head down, eyes red, and tears were flowing down her cheeks. She couldn't speak and would not raise her head to acknowledge our presence.

I had no choice but to go inside her room and check her temperature. I told her that we were very sorry and that she and her husband would be in our thoughts and prayers.

We wanted to hug her. I have never seen anyone that needed a hug more than she did, but we couldn't take the risk of infecting her since we were in close contact with many other guests. I also have never seen anyone that looked so fragile and alone. It was obvious she had never been in a situation like this before.

As we continued performing our required tasks, we couldn't help but think about her and what a long and draining ride it would be for her. The thoughts going through her mind during that two-hour ride must have been the longest ride of her life. The images of her and her husband, along with 1,000s of other passengers having the time of their lives on the cruise ships, only to be blindsided by this horrible pandemic, stayed with us that day.

We got into a routine. We donned on PPE, checked temps, doffed off PPE, and provided a briefing to the medical task force team members as well as the command staff in the command center.

For two weeks, our world was small. It consisted of spending the day on the military base and then going directly to a local hotel down the road. Because we were currently working for a Federal task force and due to the COVID uncertainty, we did not participate in any other activities. We were essentially living in a bubble of sorts.

We were lucky to watch most of the passengers get the good news that they would be leaving the compound and returning home. It was a mixture of feelings. Many of them admitted to being spoiled with everyone catering to their needs, but they were also excited to get back home in their own beds and see hometown family and friends.

Large buses were brought in to transport them to the airport. We waved good-bye as they drove away. It looked and felt more like a trip for senior high-school students headed to the beach to celebrate their senior class summer trip, than a busload of middle-aged and older individuals celebrating their trip to go home.

Since the passengers were now off of the military compound, our tasks were complete and our deployment was quickly ending. We spent a day demobilizing. After finalizing the necessary paperwork, I headed to the airport. I was assigned the team van, so I was responsible for returning it to the rental car company. This was my first exposure to how much the world we lived in just a few weeks ago had changed so much.

I arrived at the parking garage and there was no space to park. It was a ghost town. I finally found one person in the massive garage. He said to keep the van where it was. I advised him the sign said to return the vehicles in another part of the garage, but I couldn't get to it since there were vacant cars blocking all entrances.

He said he has never seen anything like this and they didn't have any more room to park all of the rental cars. With a concerned look in his eyes, he said, "Yeah, whatever is happening is going to kill our business." I just looked at him, and really didn't have the words to respond. And frankly, I didn't have a clear understanding of how his statement would become a reality.

I made my way through the garage to the ground floor. I walked a short distance to the bus stop area. This bus will take me and others to the airport. It again was eerily vacant. There were only three people that got on the bus with me.

As we rode to the airport, I looked out the window. This is San Diego, California during springtime and during summer break. The roads and sidewalks should be full of cars and people. They were empty.

I arrived at the airport with a mask and gloves on. I checked in and walked to my gate. The plane arrived a short time later. As I entered the plane, I found my seat. The airline personnel conducted their customary procedures. I looked around and noticed something I have never experienced before.

It is a large jet-liner. My guess was that it normally carries 300-400 people, but there are approximately 15-20 people on the plane. I had a window seat, and decided to move to an area where I could lay down and take a nap. I had a large section of the plane to myself. This was the third thing I saw today that proved that our world had changed.

The flight home was the smoothest and easiest flight I have ever been on. We landed and arrived at the enormous Atlanta-Hartsfield International Airport. It is a city within a city. I have traveled through this airport many times. It is always crowed with people as it is a facility servicing millions of guests and passengers every year. The reality of how much our world truly changed hit me when I walked through the Atlanta airport. It was a ghost-town. I can't emphasize how unusual it was walking through the large hallways with no people, no stores open, no personnel, no announcements; nothing.

My friend picked me up at the airport. We traveled through the city of Atlanta. I saw one last confirmation on this day that things in our world were forever changed. Atlanta is infamous for its congestion and traffic jams. But it was not on this day. The interstate highways and side streets are strangely vacant. Honestly, it was refreshing to travel through the city so quickly and easily, but it was still a reminder that whatever was happening paralyzing two famous cities to a complete halt.

I arrived home and got several calls and emails from family and friends. They asked me for my advice on what to do. I tell them this is serious and it is something that is not going to go away anytime soon. I share with them self-protection actions –wear masks and gloves, use hand cleaner, keep any shoes you wear outside the home, remove clothing as soon as you get home, and wash your hair.

Our task force typically deals with death and destruction. And although the deployment was in response to a very serious virus, it was actually a good and positive experience. We met and spent time with folks from all over the country and from all walks of life. It was the perfect example of how these extraordinary circumstances brought a diverse group of individuals together. The other task force members and I did what we could to make the best of the situation for each other and for the guests. Although we do not know the outcome or the status of these guests when they returned home, it was a privilege to help them during their time with us.

Since that time, I have had family and friends who have contracted the virus. At the writing of this story, all of them have made a complete recovery. Some have experienced more symptoms than others, but fortunately none lost their lives.

Also, I have received the COVID vaccine. My reaction to it has been typical. My arm was sore for a couple of days. The first day I felt a little flushed a few times. The second day I had no symptoms. The third day, I was lethargic and achy. I rested all day. After the third day, I had no symptoms and it didn't slow me down at all.

After receiving the vaccine, I felt a little bit of relief. I'm very healthy with no underlying medical conditions. I have taken all of the necessary steps to protect myself, my family and others. However, with the vaccine, I feel that I can somewhat participate in normal things, such as going back to the gym, etc. I still take measures such as wearing a mask and social distancing. I feel that the vaccine gives me a little bit of insurance and a better chance of fighting the virus if I do get it.

In summary, compared to other individuals and families, I have been very lucky. Overall, my COVID experience has been a positive one. However, seeing how devastating this virus has been and how it has literally destroyed families and millions of lives, I'm just so grateful and thankful, but my heartfelt sympathy goes to those so affected by this historical event.

My hope is that as bad as this whole pandemic has been, there are positive things that will come out of this. We all are realizing the reality that life is so important and so fragile. Hopefully people will appreciate each other more, regardless of our differences. We all have the same needs – a need for a home, family, friends, a job, love and respect more now than ever with this virus. I am grateful for my experiences, family and friends. We will get through this.

February Developments in 2020

By February 11th, the WHO names the coronavirus COVID-19. Ten days later, the CDC changed the criteria for counting confirmed cases and starts to track two groups: those returning to the U.S. Department of State and those identified by the U. S. Public Health network.

The last week of February, the NIH began to evaluate the safety and effectiveness of several drugs to treat COVID like the antiviral drug **remdesivir**. An American evacuated from the *Diamond Princess* Cruise ship was the first trial candidate.

Vice President Mike Pence was put in charge of the government response to COVID amidst growing criticism of the handling of the virus by the President. A patient in Washington State died marking the first U. S. death from COVID.

At about the same time CDC officials identified the first coronavirus case in the U.S. of *unknown origin* in California. This would be referred to as the first possible community spread case in the U.S.

The second week of March brought the announcement by President Trump that travel was restricted from Europe to the United States for 30 days to try to slow the virus. This ban did not apply to U. S. citizens and permanent residents who were screening before entering the U. S. At the same time the President declared a *"national emergency to free up $50 billion in federal resources to combat coronavirus."* Within days he signed a relief package including free testing for COVID-19 and paid emergency leave.

United States Interest Rates Dropped

In early March, the Federal Reserve cut interest rates by half a percentage point in an attempt to help the U.S. economy amid concerns about the virus. It was the first cut since 2008. Rates continued to drop over the course of the next year reaching a low in March of 2021 with many folks re-financing their homes to reduce the monthly payments. With the Federal Reserve rate at 0% to .25%; refinancing homes, after mortgage companies' added fees, became about 3% depending upon the applicant's financial background; overall a nice reduction in mortgage payments.

Responses from Around the World

Every country dealt with the virus in different ways. **Iran** temporarily released 54,000 prisoners and deployed hundreds of thousands of health workers to contain the virus. This occurring while 23 members of Iran's parliament tested positive on March 3rd.

The largest outbreak in Europe was in **Italy**'s Lombardy region. That area had a complete lockdown in effect which affected about 100,000 people during the last week of February. By March 8th, the Italian Prime Minister Giuseppe Conte placed travel restrictions on the entire Lombardy region and 14 other provinces, restricting the movements of more than 10 million people in the northern part of Italy. By March 9th he locked down the entire country.

China downplayed the virus by announcing on March 19th that there were no new locally transmitted cases for the first time. Few believed the numbers coming out of China which were exceptionally low.

By the third week of March the United Nations called for an immediate global ceasefire in order to deal with the pandemic. The International Olympic Committee president Thomas Bach postponed the Olympics until 2021. The pandemic was affecting us all, globally. Some caught the virus and others escaped it.

Mark 11:22-24 - And Jesus answered them, "Have faith in God. Truly, I say to you, whoever says to this mountain, 'Be taken up and thrown into the sea,' and does not doubt in his heart, but believes that what he says will come to pass, it will be done for him. Therefore I tell you, whatever you ask in prayer, believe that you have received it, and it will be yours.

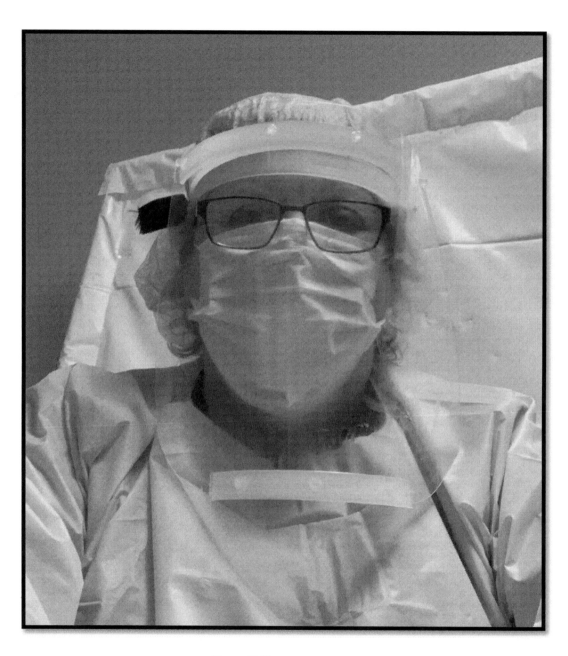

Figure 10 Nurse.

Chapter 2

Personal Experiences

Contact, Many not Symptomatic

An article, by Tim Richards, as told to Brooke Nelson, described how one patient got the virus: "My wife, Megan, and I went out to dinner with an old friend who we had not seen in a while. There had been some talk of COVID-19 in the news, but it was early in the outbreak and people were still going about their daily routines. Even though everyone in our group felt perfectly fine, we took precautions: We washed our hands with soap and used hand sanitizer, did not share food, and had no significantly close contact."

He went on to say, "A few days later, our friend called and told us that she had tested positive for the coronavirus. She had felt some mild symptoms for a day or so after the dinner and was able to be tested because she is a doctor. Despite our precautions that night, the virus was also passed to me and another friend who had joined us. That makes two people who caught the virus from someone with no symptoms or reason to believe she had the virus."

"We are not the only ones." In a study published on MedRx iv about the COVID-19 outbreaks abroad, researchers found that 48 percent of cases in Singapore and 62 percent of cases in Tianjin, China, could be linked to people who were pre-symptomatic, or had not developed symptoms yet. (The study has not yet been peer-reviewed.) That's why the U.S. Centers for Disease Control and Prevention (CDC) has recommended reducing physical contact with others and limiting group gatherings to ten people, even if you do not feel sick. (March 26, 2020).

Sheltering in Place – Brunswick County[23]

By Shawn Russell, Sunset Harbor, NC

Early Indications

The year 2020 started with much controversy and turmoil. The biggest news of the day was the impeachment of President Donald Trump. The trial had occupied the news for months. Everyone was sick of it, yet, we had to suffer through that entire political circus. The President was acquitted by the Senate on February 5th and at the same time a story beneath the fold of the newspapers concerned a virus and possible pandemic out of China. Not many in America were concerned at the time as most of our leaders dismissed it.

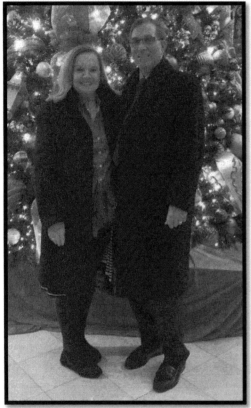

Figure 11 Tom & Mary Shawn Russell.

The first indication we had that all was not right in America occurred for my family when in mid-February my husband's prescription medication, Losartan, could not be filled by Express Scripts Home Delivery. When we inquired as to why, it was revealed that the medication was "not available." When we continued to investigate why the drug was not available, we were told that because it was made in China. Obviously, the story that the coronavirus from China was nothing to worry about was more serious than was being portrayed in early to mid-February. Also, troubling was the fact that China controlled America's pharmaceutical production. How could America allow that to happen? Who sold out such a critical industry to a country that is a world competitor at best and an enemy at worst?

February 14th was another signal that the virus was more of a threat than we were originally told. During my husband annual exam, an entire new check-in process had been initiated. Questions about travel both outside the country and outside the county were asked. Questions about recent sicknesses were also asked prior to meeting with the doctor.

---

[23] Sheltering in Place – Brunswick County. By Mary Shawn Russell, Sunset Harbor, North Carolina. May 7, 2020.

This started to really trouble us. Would this get worse? How far were they going to go concerning the invasion of our privacy and possibly our freedoms. The closest alligator to our boat was our upcoming trip to Pensacola, Florida for our nephew's wedding and a follow-on trip to Naples, Florida just a couple weeks away.

Increased Anxiety – Changing Behavior

Despite the quarantine of a Carnival Cruise ship in early February and the first reported death in America from the disease, there was increased anxiety but no restrictions to travel; so, we departed for our nephew's wedding in Florida. We couldn't help but to think about the news of the virus and believe it was in the background of everyone's mind at the wedding. There were no restrictions for social distancing and the shaking of hands as family member gathered for this grand celebration was never a second thought. Also interesting was the fact that our nephew that was wed was a doctor just finishing up his internship and his new bride, was a nurse.

We proceeded to Naples, Florida for fourteen days of fun and relaxation on March 8th. Shortly thereafter President Trump issued a national emergency. This was now getting everyone's attention. The Center for Disease Control warned against holding large gatherings of over 50 people. We decided that this virus was spiraling out of control so we decided to cut our trip short and return to North Carolina. It really hit home for us in a rest stop in Georgia, when my husband washed his hands. Another patron approached my husband coughing and hacking throughout the facility. We discontinued the use of state operated rest areas and relied on Travel Centers like Pilot or Loves. We started washing our hands every time we touched a foreign object (gas pumps, door handles, etc.). Clearly, this virus had already changed the way we conducted our lives before the government came in and controlled our lives for us.

Heavy Hand of Government

By the time we had returned from Florida the Governor of North Carolina had issued an Executive Order declaring a State of Emergency. He so ordered all non-essential citizens to shelter in place, conduct separation of at least six feet (social distancing) and the closure of all non-essential businesses. Everyone bought into the plan for it was only to last two weeks and it was to help our hospitals from being overwhelmed (flatten the curve they called it). Most everyone thought that they were doing their civic duty and could last two weeks. Not many folks thought that it could last three months nor did they sign up for their rights to be trampled on indefinitely by a government that clearly was moving the goal posts to justify the closure. Models were presented daily that projected the deaths and hospitalized. These projections that the American public saw never came close to reality, in my opinion. Many started to question the Center for Disease Control and trust became an issue. Protest rallies were conducted in Raleigh as businesses went bankrupt and had to close. The Federal Government spent trillions of dollars to help keep business from bankruptcy and employees from going on unemployment. Yet, over 30 million filed for unemployment in one week's time. Every tax-paying citizen was given $1,200 and child

$500 from the federal government to hold them over. This check did not come close to the losses taken from the closures and 30% drop in the stock market.

Sheltering in Place

For my family, the biggest changes were social. Everyone was wracked with fear as to who had the virus and who did not. Social media and the phone became the primary way to communicate. I spent hours on the phone with my sister on more than one occasion, as there was not a lot else to do. Shopping was limited to the local grocery store which had limited items. The toilet paper ran out early as did most canned foods. Fresh vegetables were plentiful but as the meat packing plants became centers for the virus, meat products had to be rationed. Government regulations required only a certain number of shoppers in grocery and home improvement stores based on square footage. The Walmart Greeter became the person who told you when you could go in to shop. Lines formed outside the stores that were allowed to be open. Some stores provided sanitized wipe down towelettes; some did not.

We cooked more at home as restaurants were only allowed to operate their drive through window or take out service. We attempted to frequent our local restaurants to keep them open often utilizing Jersey Mikes, Subway, McDonalds, and Bojangles. Mostly comfort food. We quickly tired of eating in the car, as if we were still in our youth going to the drive-in. Those restaurants where you had to go inside for take-out, placed feet markings on the floor which depicted where you were to stand and to maintain the required six-foot social separation from other patrons. Check-out counters were separated by plexi-glass barriers to help keep the virus/germs from the cashier.

During our time in "shelter in place" we utilized our home gym extensively. My husband rode his bike, though not with his biking club buddies as they cancelled all their weekly group rides. I continued my photography and posted my photos on Facebook to provide my friends hope that we will survive this.

Our $2,400 ($1,200 per citizen) stimulus check arrived into our checking account in March but was quickly spent on a new washer and dryer. It took some research to find a washer and dryer to purchase that was not made in China. By this point we started looking at labels and were determined to by nothing from China, who had inflicted this disease on the world. Most thought that China had the opportunity to tell the truth about the virus early on and protect its spread to the world but did not do so.

As April came and went, the shelter-in-place order and closure of the economy in North Carolina was extended until May 8th. Everyone started to question the state government. Why were some businesses allowed to stay open and others were not allowed to open their business? Some of these orders made absolutely no sense to many. To be able to worship in a church during the Easter Holiday was a big issue…not allowed. Churches transitioned to preaching via social media. Some churches utilized parking lot drive-in movie type services. Worshipers remained in their cars while the minister preached over a loud speaker.

Each state developed their own plans to reopen their economies. On paper it looked like those with Republican governors were opening the fastest while those states with Democrat governors were delaying their openings. This appearance looked like dirty politics during a national election year. The American citizenry became more mistrustful of government/politics and angry. As the government ordered shutdown continued month-after-month, citizen thinking started to change. They desired to go back to work. They wanted to be responsible for protecting their own health and let government protect their freedoms. These people were opposed to the government responsible for their health and trampling their freedoms.

Second Order Effects

Having lived through this period was not without its advances. We learned how to defeat a virus by washing our hands frequently, wearing a mask, social distancing, not shaking hands, and carrying disinfectant spray in all our cars to clean after we touched any foreign object.

Another good thing that the coronavirus brought to America was the lack of junk mail. All that daily postage that normally ends up in the "circular file" was almost non-existent.

Conclusion

The coronavirus exposed the character and creative ingenuity of the American people. Americans stepped up and banded together to meet this invisible enemy without the protections required preventing infection. We all had one huge thing in common... *The Coronavirus.* Most did their duty as citizens to protect themselves and each other. Neighbors helped neighbors. Now, it is time to slowly step back into our regular lives as we knew it and reopen this great nation.

Getting Tested

The general public of the U. S. found it difficult to get a COVID test. Unless a person had close contact with another infected person or were in the hospital they could not get a test. The first week of March, the CDC removed these earlier restrictions and allowed health workers to use their own judgment to determine if signs and symptoms warranted a test.

When first experiencing symptoms patients attempted to get a COVID - 19 test. Initially, medical personnel were administering a flu test first, to determine if those symptoms were the flu. If the flu test came back negative, then a COVID test was conducted. Slowly, the practice became...if you have mild symptoms stay at home and only come to the emergency rooms or doctor's office if having difficulty breathing. Then, an appointment was needed and patients were advised to call their doctor or emergency room to determine IF they should come in. Slowly, medical tests and drive in testing sites were announced and COVID patients were kept away from the interior of hospitals in order to protect other patients and staff. Unnecessary surgeries were postponed and people were generally advised to not come to the hospitals unless medical care was absolutely needed.

Testing was generally limited to those who had a fever and had been exposed to another positive patient or had traveled outside of the United States. Some wanting testing, were denied. As the understanding of the virus grew, testing practices grew; varying in different parts of the country.

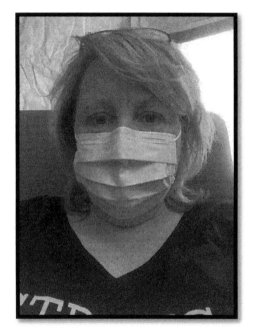

Jennifer Fisher Tried to Get Tested

Figure 12 Jennifer Fisher attempting to get a COVID test.

Jennifer Fisher of Stedman, NC went to nearby Cape Fear Valley Hospital in Fayetteville, NC early-March 2020 asking for a Coronavirus test. Her symptoms were fever, sore throat, headache and a general extreme tiredness. She was denied a test. "It was very confusing, based upon all the information provided in the news which encouraged people to get tested. It made me wonder how many individuals actually had the virus and were not being tested," she said. Later she realized that she most likely *did* have the virus, in addition to her husband, Jonathan, who had similar symptoms. She went home, self-isolated for 14 days and eventually recovered.

In February, about two weeks earlier, her son, Isaih Fisher, 14 years old, and a freshman at Cape Fear High School, had fallen sick. He was extremely fatigued and could not get out of bed. He had a bad headache, sore throat and was vomiting. On a scale of 1 to 10, he rated his illness 8 or 9…the worst he had ever had. This *straight A student*, missed school for nine days, very ill. He was taken to the doctor's office at the time and given a flu test, which came back negative. This was prior to the school closing. And it was prior to having access for a COVID test, even with symptoms, unless you have traveled out of country or been exposed to COVID, for *sure*.

When Jennifer Fisher, the mom, got sick, she had a sore throat, headache fatigue, and vomiting, but with mild symptoms. Even though she requested testing, Jennifer Fisher was not given either flu or a coronavirus test.   Jonathan, the father, had headache, fatigue, and sore throat also; no test given. COVID-19 counts did not include this family. Add three more to Cumberland County, North Carolina. How many others had this experience?

During her illness, while self-quarantining, several members of the community supported her family by bringing meals and handmade masks to her doorstep. She would wave at them through the window, thanking them. "It made me feel loved by our family and friends. Luckily, none of them got it," she said. The two younger sons in the family, Elijah, 9 years old, and Jacob, 12 years old, seemingly escaped the disease.

This was early in the process when only those with known connections to another COVID patient were tested; or if the person had traveled outside of the United States.

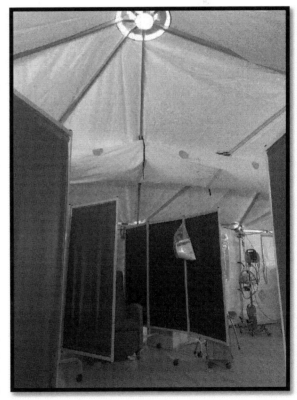

Figure 13 Cape Fear Valley COVID screening tent outside of the main hospital.

The COVID screening tent outside of the main hospital at Cape Fear Valley Hospital, Fayetteville, North Carolina is shown. It was denying testing but obviously empty.

Getting Admitted

Those who tested positive (and somehow actually got a test to prove it) or had breathing difficulties were usually admitted into hospitals. In some areas, special facilities were set up to specifically handle the COVID cases in order to try to contain the virus. These ranged from sports arenas to Navy ships like the *Comfort and Mercy*. These hospital ships were quickly set up with one thousand beds each and fully staffed with medical personnel. Nurses and doctors awaited the onset of peaks where the most populated patients resided. At first New York and California (the *Comfort* arrived in New York harbor on March 27, 2020) were noted to need these beds with the Mayor of New York begging for assistance. They were provided to care for the regular patients so the hospitals could have space for the COVID patients.

Throughout the outbreak in New York City and surrounding Burroughs, Mayor Andrew Cuomo and President Trump exchanged jabs on the news media as the Mayor continually asked for supplies. President Trump continued to supply those supplies, particularly thousands of ventilators. At one point, Mayor Cuomo asked for 40,000 ventilators for patients, in addition to the stockpiles they had in the city and state. In the end, he did not need that many. In the end he never used the Navy ships. In the end Cuomo made decisions to send the sick to nursing homes which ultimately caused death rates in those facilities to rise; later questioned as to the numbers of death which may have been inaccurately reported at the time. By March 2021, his own staff members accused him of sexual harassment and cases remain open as of June 2021.

President Trump responded to growing needs for ventilators and personal protective equipment by asking manufacturers around the country to shut down regular operations and begin manufacturing ventilators; which quickly happened. Many businesses re-directed their factories and personnel and made ventilators, masks, gowns, gloves and other medical supplies while the pandemic victims grew.

Initially Washington state was the *hotspot*, as they were known; the first large outbreak in the United States; primarily nursing homes there. But they soon got a handle on the viral patients and did not need additional beds.

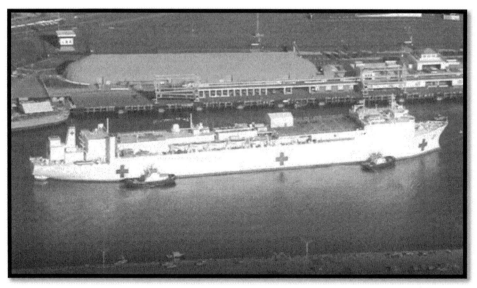

Figure 14 The Naval Ship, USNS Mercy, arriving in the port of Los Angeles, CA.[24]

---

[24] Aerial view of the Hospital ship USNS Mercy docked at Naval Base San Diego on March 20, 2020 in San Diego, California. California (Photo by Sean M. Haffey/Getty Images)

Navy Ship Mercy Arrives in the Port of LA - to Help Hospitals Strained by Coronavirus[25]

The 1,000-bed hospital ship, named in the spirit of compassion, will treat non-COVID-19 patients, allowing land-based hospitals to devote resources to the fast-spreading virus.

Southern California's hospitals received some much-needed relief in the battle against the new coronavirus when an oil tanker that was converted into a floating 1,000-bed hospital arrived Friday morning in the Port of Los Angeles.

USNS Mercy departed Naval Station San Diego Monday and entered the Port of Los Angeles at about 8:15 a.m. to dock at the cruise ship terminal. Non-COVID-19 patients will be treated on the hospital ship, part of a plan to free up land-based hospitals to respond to the coronavirus crisis.

The ship's medical crew includes Commander Edgar San Luis, of Long Beach. "It feels like I'm coming back home," San Luis said. "It brings me great joy to be a part of something of this magnitude, to help the city of Los Angeles. Being born and raised, in Los Angeles it brings it closer to home for me to serve the population of LA."

There will be a gradual transfer of patients to the ship from land-based hospitals, as needed. "It brings me great joy to be a part of something of this magnitude to help the city of Los Angeles," he says. Hetty Chang reports for the NBC4 News at 11 p.m. Mar. 26, 2020.

At a midday news conference with the giant ship as a backdrop, Gov. Gavin Newsom thanked the administration of President Trump for its support and timely response to the state's urgent medical needs. California reported a 26-percent increase in COVID-19 cases on Thursday. "We are seeing a spike that we were preparing for," Newsom said.

…"This global crisis demands whole of government response, and we are ready to support," said Navy Capt. John Rotruck, Mercy's military treatment facility commanding officer. "Mercy brings a team of medical professionals; medical equipment and supplies, all of which will act, in essence, as a `relief valve' for local civilian hospitals in Los Angeles so that local health professionals can better focus on COVID-19 cases.

"We will use our agility and responsiveness as an afloat medical treatment facility to do what the country asks, and bring relief where we are needed most."

---

[25] NBC Los Angeles news. Jonathan Lloyd and Hetty Chang • Published March 27, 2020 • Updated on March 27, 2020 at 2:04 pm. https://www.nbclosangeles.com/news/coronavirus/coronavirus-COVID-19-navy-hospital-ship-mercy-los-angeles-california/2336306/

At full capacity, Mercy will be the largest hospital in Los Angeles.

"This will be a COVID-19-free bubble," said Los Angeles Mayor Eric Garcetti, who served as an intelligence officer in the United States Navy Reserve. "Every bed not taken in Los Angeles… will mean one more bed for the surge the governor spoke about. This truly is Mercy on the water."

The current USNS Mercy is the third Navy ship to carry the name, signifying compassion. The first was built as Saratoga in 1907 and served as an Army troop transport during World War I. It was renamed Mercy and converted to a hospital ship. Commissioned in January 1918, the first Mercy completed four round trips to France and carried nearly 2,000 casualties. The second Mercy was commissioned in August 1944.

USNS Comfort Will Depart for New York on Saturday with Trump, Modly in Attendance[26]   **By Megan Eckstein   March 26, 2020**

Supplies and personnel are loaded aboard the Military Sealift Command hospital ship USNS Comfort (T-AH 20) at Naval Station Norfolk, Va., March 24, 2020. Comfort is preparing to deploy in support of the nation's COVID-19 response efforts and will serve as a referral hospital for non-COVID-19 patients currently admitted to shore-based hospitals. This allows shore-based hospitals to focus their efforts on COVID-19 cases.

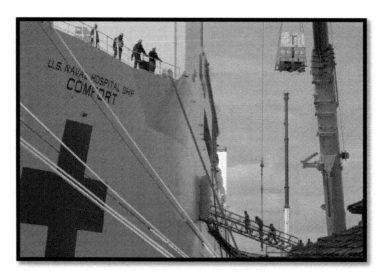

Figure 15 US Navy Photo.

---

[26] USNI News. Eckstein, Megan. https://news.usni.org/2020/03/26/usns-comfort-departs-for-new-york-on-saturday-with-trump-modly-in-attendance. March 26, 2020.

Supplies and personnel are loaded aboard the Military Sealift Command hospital ship USNS Comfort (T-AH 20) at Naval Station Norfolk, Va., March 24, 2020. US Navy photo.

The Pentagon – Hospital ship USNS Comfort (T-AH-20) will leave for New York City on Saturday, with President Donald Trump and Acting Secretary of the Navy Thomas Modly on hand to see off the ship from Naval Station, Norfolk, Va.

Trump announced today he would travel to Norfolk on Saturday "to bid bon voyage to the hospital ship USNS Comfort (T-AH-20) as it leaves for New York City to the frontlines of the COVID-19 virus response. The USNS Comfort will sail well ahead of its originally scheduled departure time to answer America's call to battle against the global pandemic here at home," reads a White House news release.

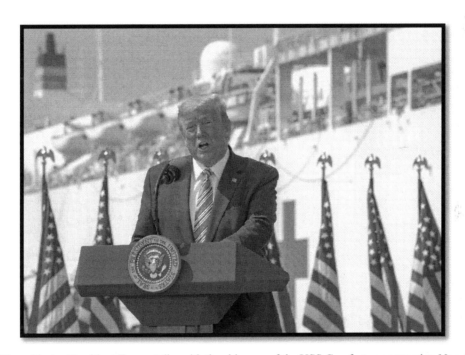

Figure 16 US Navy Photo. President Trump talks with the shipman of the USS Comfort upon travel to New York.

"As we gathered today, our country is at war with an invisible enemy. We are marshaling the full power of the American nation, economic, scientific, medical and military to vanquish the virus," Trump said standing on the pier with *Comfort* in the background.[27]

"The crew of the Navy hospital ship, *USNS Comfort*, which is really something, will embark for New York City where they will join the ranks of tens of thousands of amazing

---

[27] USNI News. https://news.usni.org/2020/03/28/trump-gives-usns-comfort-a-send-off-as-hospital-ship-departs-for-new-york.

doctors, nurses, and medical professionals who are battling to save American lives. This great ship behind me is a 70,000-ton message of hope and solidarity to the incredible people of New York."[28]

According to Trump, "the ship is set to arrive at the Norwegian Cruise Line terminal at Pier 90 in Manhattan on Monday and begin seeing patients on Tuesday."[29]

Earlier in the day, Modly said in a Pentagon press briefing that "we've accelerated the plan for Comfort. We had originally been looking at April 3, but in all likelihood, she's going to be getting underway this weekend. So hopefully she'll be there in New York by the early part of next week."

The hospital ship, a converted San Clemente-class super tanker that has provided global medical support under the Military Sealift Command for 33 years, was undergoing maintenance work in Norfolk when Trump announced the ship would be deployed to support New York's COVID-19 outbreak. Comfort will not take on infected patients but will rather care for patients with other needs – emergency surgeries, trauma care and more – to free up beds and doctors at New York hospitals so they can deal with the virus.

Comfort's sister ship, USNS Mercy (T-AH-19), departed San Diego on Monday and should pull into Los Angeles tomorrow, after at-sea training and ballasting this week.

The White House statement adds that "over 1,200 medical personnel and critical supplies will be onboard the vessel. They will bring to bear the skills, care, and compassion needed to wage this fight against an invisible enemy. These doctors, nurses, anesthesiologists, x-ray technicians, orderlies, and other medical staff will augment and support New York City's medical community and conserve hospital capacity by treating some non-COVID-19 patients aboard the USNS Comfort."

The nation worked together. The military, small and large businesses, manufacturing plants, and individuals brought the ingenuity and resources together to fight this virus.

———

Ephesians 2:8-9 - For by grace you have been saved through faith. And this is not your own doing; it is the gift of God, not a result of works, so that no one may boast.

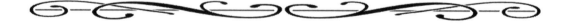

[28] IBID.
[29] IBID.

Chapter 3

The Plan to Re-Open America

President Trumps Plan to Reopen America[30]

Daily, the television carries the message from the Task Force Committee and the President of the United State, Donald J. Trump. Regardless of political opinion, it is reassuring and helpful to touch base with the American public and keep them apprised of the latest U. S. research and logic for mitigating the virus.

The Plan[31]

The plan provides governors across the nation a road map for recovering from the economic pain of the coronavirus pandemic, laying out "a phased and deliberate approach" to restoring normal activity in places that have strong testing and are seeing a decrease in COVID-19 cases.

"We're starting our life again," Trump said during his daily press briefing. "We're starting rejuvenation of our economy again." He added, "This is a gradual process."

The new guidelines are aimed at easing restrictions in areas with low transmission of the coronavirus, while holding the line in harder-hit locations. They make clear that the return to normalcy will be a far longer process than Trump initially envisioned, with federal officials warning that some social distancing measures may need to remain in place through the end of the year to prevent a new outbreak. And they largely reinforce the plans already under development by governors, who have the primary responsibility for public health in their states.

"You're going to call your own shots," Trump told the governors Thursday afternoon in a conference call, according to an audio recording obtained by The Associated Press. "We're going to be standing alongside of you."

---

[30] https://kfor.com/health/coronavirus/read-president-trumps-three-step-plan-to-reopen-americas-economy-during-coronavirus-crisis/
[31] IBID.

Places with declining infections and strong testing would begin a three-phase gradual reopening of businesses and schools.

Phase One

In Phase One, the plan recommended strict social distancing for all people in public. Gatherings larger than 10 people are to be avoided and nonessential travel is discouraged.

Phase Two

In Phase Two, people are encouraged to maximize social distancing where possible and limit gatherings to no more than 50 people unless precautionary measures are taken. Travel could resume.

Phase Three

Phase Three envisions a return to normalcy for most Americans, with a focus on identification and isolation of any new infections.

Governors of both parties made clear they will move at their own pace.

Delaware Gov. John Carney, a Democrat, said the guidelines "seem to make sense.""We're days, maybe weeks away from the starting line and then you have to have 14 days of declining cases, of declining symptoms and hospital capacity that exists in case you have a rebound," he said.

West Virginia Gov. Jim Justice, a Trump ally, cautiously floated the idea of reopening parts of the state, but said testing capacity and contact tracing would need to be considerably ramped up before restrictions could be safely lifted."All would be forgotten very quickly if we moved into a stage quicker than we should, and then we got into a situation where we had people dying like flies," Justice told reporters.

At earliest, the guidelines suggest, some parts of the country could see a resumption in normal commerce and social gatherings after a month of evaluating whether easing up on restrictions has led to a resurgence in virus cases. In other parts of the country, or if virus cases pick up, it could be substantially longer.

In briefing the governors on the plan, Trump said they were going to be responsible for deciding when it is safe to lift restrictions in their states. Just days before, he had drawn swift pushback for claiming he had the absolute authority to determine how and when states reopen.

"We have a very large number of states that want to get going and they're in very good shape," Trump said. "That's good with us, frankly."

Those most susceptible to the respiratory disease are advised to remain sheltered in place until their area enters the final phase – and even encouraged to take precautions to avoid close contact with other people.

Governors, for their part, had been moving ahead with their own plans for how to safely revive normal activity. Seven Midwestern governors announced Thursday they will coordinate on reopening their economies. Similar pacts were announced earlier in the week in the West and Northeast.

Two in three Americans expressed concerns that restrictions meant to slow the spread of the virus would be eased too quickly, according to a Pew Research Center survey released Thursday.

Trump also held conference calls Thursday with lawmakers he named to a new congressional advisory task force on reviving the economy. The economic costs were clear in new federal data showing that at least 22 million Americans have been thrown out of work in the last month. But the legislators repeatedly urged the president not to sacrifice public health by moving too quickly.

"My highest priority on this task force will be to ensure the federal government's efforts to reopen our economy are bipartisan, data-driven, and based on the expertise of public health professionals," said Democratic Sen. Mark Warner of Virginia.

The federal government envisions a gradual recovery from the virus, in which disruptive mitigation measures may be needed in some places at least until a vaccine is available – a milestone unlikely to be reached until sometime next year.

"It's not going to immediately be a situation where we have stadiums full of people," said Housing and Urban Development Secretary Ben Carson on Thursday. "We're Americans. We will adapt," he added.

Trump on Thursday claimed the U.S. has "built the most advanced and robust testing anywhere in the world." But even people close to him warned more would be necessary.

"We are struggling with testing at a large scale," said South Carolina Sen. Lindsey Graham. "You really can't go back to work until we have more tests."

But some of Trump's conservative allies, like economist Stephen Moore, have encouraged him to act swiftly, warning of "a mini Great Depression if we keep the economy shut down."

"That is a catastrophic outcome for our country. Period," Moore said he advised the president. "We can't have 30 million people in this country unemployed or you're going to have social chaos."

A big testing ground for Trump's road map could be Texas, where Republican Gov. Greg Abbott, who has stuck close to federal guidance throughout the crisis, will lay out his reopening plan Friday. Abbott has said the process will be gradual, but he is facing pressure from conservative lawmakers to get Texas back to work.

———————————

Many questions remained on the minds of the regular folks. When would we be able to go shopping again? How about a restaurant sit-down meal? We waited patiently for how each state will respond and when we can ease our restrictive movements.

By May 2021, it was still unclear when everything would be open and masks no longer required. For a while, in the spring of 2021, officials hinted at an opening by July 4th, but that is being doubted by many at this time. Time will tell.

State Restrictions

State restrictions varied by state in 2020 depending upon the impact of the COVID-19 virus. Many mirrored those in North Carolina (those without huge impacts.)

NC State Restrictions and Executive Orders by the Governor

Executive Order 117: Restricted mass gatherings of ten or more people

Executive Order 121: Stay at Home Order issued by Governor Roy Cooper, which began on March 30th at 5 p.m. until April 29th, 2020. It was later extended to May 8th.

This order directed people to stay home except to visit essential businesses, exercise outdoors, or help a family member. It specifically banned the gathering of more than ten people and directs social distancing of six feet apart.

Executive Order 131 addressed three specific issues:

It required retail stores that are still operating to implement new social distancing policies to make shopping safer for customer and employees. It made COVID-19 guidelines mandatory for nursing facilities, and recommended other long-term care facilities to do the same. It also sped up the process to get benefits to people who are unemployed.

Brunswick County, NC State of Emergency Declaration

While every state in the nation had been approved for a Declaration of a State of Emergency, most counties followed. Brunswick County Commission Chairman Frank

Williams issued the state of emergency due to the COVID-19 on Tuesday, March 24, 2020. This declaration covers all incorporated sections of the county. The Government County offices remained open but with many adaptations such as making an appointment ahead of time and special handling with reasonable restrictions. By the end of March in 2021, now Chairman of the Brunswick County Commission, Randy Thompson, cancelled the county state of emergency as numbers of residents with COVID were drastically reduced to less than 300 in the county.

Interestingly, all the county and state restrictions did not include restrictions or prohibitions involving evacuations, curfews, alcohol, or weapons.

May 2020

As of May 1, 2020, the states were given the direction by the White House Corona Virus Task Force, to create plans to Open Back-Up America. Phases of opening were recommended, all tied to statistical data and Governors were asked to adapt them for their own circumstances. This was later to become quite a challenge for some states. Some chose to open totally and others stayed locked down for much longer periods of time. Schools were closed and life was indeed not normal. Even by March of 2021, schools were not open full time and some not at all continuing virtual learning on laptop computers.

The Stimulus Package and Coronavirus Relief Bills

By the 23rd of April Congress appropriated more funding for America to assist in recovering from the virus hardships caused by the shut-down of businesses and unemployment of the U.S. worker. There was also a lot of discussion about funding for the states and cities. Amidst the discussions of this bill, is whether to spend the money we do not presently have, taking it from future generations.

The first of several stimulus bills was signed by Congress to offset the economic damage caused by the corona virus for a cost of $2 trillion dollars. Almost every adult U. S. citizen would receive a check for $600. President Trump signed this stimulus package into law on March 27th. Later in December of 2020, another check was in the making for $1200 and once again in March of 2021 another check for $1400. The U. S. government at the hands of Congress was drastically increasing the national debt to aid the citizens get through all the financial hardship which ensured after businesses shut down and many lost their jobs or were put on furlough indefinitely.

The Presidents (Trump) rescue package, which included 9 trillion in stimulus funds, was aimed at helping to rebuild the economy. People were anxious to go back to work. Most were optimistic about the future. Democrats did not want a payroll tax cut, so that was not done, but the stimulus checks should have helped everyone who received them. It went something like this:

House Passes 'Interim' $484 Billion Coronavirus Relief Bill[32] April 2020

It eventually passed the house late today for small business aid, hospital aid, and the like. Small groups of lawmakers were brought into the chamber to vote, some wearing masks. Thirty-five house members did not show up for today's house vote. Excerpts of the report by the Huff Post include:

Washington — After weeks of bitter negotiations, Republicans and Democrats in Congress passed a nearly $500 billion coronavirus relief package on Thursday that will replenish the Paycheck Protection Program, which supports small businesses, and provide emergency money for hospitals. The package now goes to President Donald Trump for his signature.

Over the course of about an hour and a half, lawmakers took turns coming to the House floor to vote in groups of 40. Speaker Nancy Pelosi (D-Calif.) told representatives she wanted to avoid the usual crowds during a vote, and most lawmakers were happy to observe social distancing guidelines by quickly coming to the House chamber, inserting their voting card and then immediately leaving.

During debate of the relief package, a number of Republicans could be spotted in the House chamber without masks — and an even greater number of lawmakers seemed to take the recommended 6 foot distance between people as a mere suggestion.

The bill itself would provide $310 billion more for the Paycheck Protection Program, $60 billion in economic disaster loans for small businesses, $75 billion for hospitals and $25 billion more for coronavirus testing. The original funding dedicated to the Paycheck Protection Program, which was established in the $2.2 coronavirus relief bill that passed four weeks ago, ran dry after only two weeks — and most Republicans support emergency loans for small businesses.

Coronavirus has now killed about as many people in the U.S. in two months as there are suicides in the U.S. every year — roughly 50,000 — and coronavirus deaths increased tenfold in the past month with little sign of slowing down.

Instead, the only lawmakers who expressed frustration with the legislation — known in Congress as "Phase 3.5," because Congress has already passed three other bills and Democratic leadership had promised a larger measure for the fourth — came from the Democratic side.

Pelosi, who largely wrote the bill through negotiations with McConnell, said Congress was still in the "mitigation" phase of combating coronavirus and that additional action would be needed. And Minority Leader Kevin McCarthy (R-Calif.) said essential

---

[32] House Passes 'Interim' $484 Billion Coronavirus Relief Bill. HuffPost. Matt Fuller, Huff Post, April 23, 2020.

workers whose lives are on the line "deserve a government that strives to meet that very same level of dedication."

"That is the promise I will make," McCarthy said. "That we will bring the same dedication that you bring to help others that you don't even know."

Note: Portion of the complete article deleted were primarily related to political arguments for and against; now deemed by this author as inconsequential.

Georgia Opens Up – April 2020 – the way it was

There is word that the state of Georgia is being opened up completely. The President is not pleased with spas, beauty parlors, tattoo parlors, etc. being opened right now while the state is not following the guidelines being recommended by the White House Task Force. The President and his advisors, all agreed, the governor should do what he feels is best for Georgia. The rest of the nation holds their breath and watches to see what will happen in Georgia.

Brian Kemp, Governor of Georgia, Press Release[33]

Excerpts from: Gov. Kemp Updates. Georgians on COVID-19[34] [35]

April 20, 2020

Atlanta, GA - Today Governor Brian P. Kemp provided the following update on COVID-19 in Georgia. Governor Kemp was joined by Lieutenant Governor Geoff Duncan, Speaker David Ralston, Georgia National Guard Adjutant General Tom Carden, Georgia Department of Public Health Commissioner Kathleen Toomey, and GEMA/HS Director Homer Bryson.

"Good afternoon, everyone. Today I'm joined by Lieutenant Governor Geoff Duncan, Speaker David Ralston, General Tom Carden, Dr. Kathleen Toomey, and GEMA Director Homer Bryson."

"As of noon today, we now have 18,947 COVID-19 cases in Georgia with 733 deaths. The state lab has processed 5,362 tests, and commercial vendors have processed 78,966 tests. We understand that these are more than just numbers. These are Georgians. These are families and communities impacted. Our prayers remain with the victims and their

---

[33] Georgia Press Release. www.gdol.ga.gov. https://gov.georgia.gov/press-releases/2020-04-22/gov-kemp-georgia-dept-labor-address-unemployment-options.
[34] IBID. https://gov.georgia.gov/press-releases
[35] Director of Communications & Chief Deputy Executive Counsel
Candice Broce. candice.broce@georgia.gov. Press Secretary Cody Hall. cody.hall@georgia.gov.

loved ones. We lift up those who are battling this terrible virus. We remain focused on the safety and well-being of every person who calls Georgia home."

"Informed by the Coronavirus Task Force and public health officials, 'Opening-Up America Again' includes three phases to safely reopen and get folks back to work. To initiate Phase One, a state must meet a series of basic criteria, which can be tailored to reflect specific circumstances for a regional or statewide approach. For weeks now, our state has taken targeted action to prevent, detect, and address the spread of coronavirus by leveraging data and advice from health officials in the public and private sectors. Thanks to this methodical approach and the millions of Georgians who have worked diligently to slow the spread of coronavirus, we are on track to meet the gating criteria for Phase One."

"According to the Department of Public Health, reports of emergency room visits for flu-like illnesses are declining, documented COVID-19 cases have flattened and appear to be declining, and we have seen declining emergency room visits in general. By expanding our hospital bed capacity - including the temporary facility at the Georgia World Congress Center - we have the ability to treat patients without crisis care in hospital settings. Our proactive actions have reduced stress and strain on area hospitals as well as the communities and families that they serve."

"Now, a key component of the gating criteria is testing. For weeks, I have expressed my frustration with the status of testing and committed more resources to expansion. We partnered with the University System of Georgia, partnered with the private sector to offer drive-thru services, and recently empowered public health departments across Georgia to offer testing for all symptomatic individuals. Today we're taking this effort to the next level by announcing an even broader partnership with the state's dedicated health sciences university and its health system to double down on our testing capacity and meet the requirements necessary to move forward with the president's plan."

"As many of you know, Augusta University Health launched a telemedicine app as part of their comprehensive plan to screen, test, and treat Georgia patients through an algorithm designed by experts at the Medical College of Georgia. This app has enhanced public health while reducing exposure for our doctors, nurses, and medical staff. We are encouraging symptomatic Georgians to download the app this week and begin the screening process. ... If you begin to display symptoms consistent with COVID-19 – day or night – you can log onto AU Health's telemedicine app or call to get screened by a clinician. If you meet criteria for testing, staff will contact you to schedule a test at one of the state's designated testing locations near your home. Your healthcare information will be securely transmitted to your designated testing site."

"This streamlined process reduces stress on both the patient and testing site workers. Once you arrive for your appointment, you will provide a specimen for testing. From there, we will leverage the power of several key academic institutions in the state to process tests."

….."In the same way that we carefully closed businesses and urged operations to end to mitigate the virus' spread, today, we are announcing plans to incrementally - and safely -

reopen sectors of our economy. To help in the battle against COVID-19, healthcare facilities across Georgia voluntarily temporarily stopped elective surgeries to reduce equipment and personnel shortages. This selfless act by healthcare leaders enhanced our ability to keep Georgians safe. However, many now find themselves in a difficult financial situation, some losing millions of dollars a day as they sacrifice for the greater good. This is not sustainable long-term for these facilities. ... I believe Georgia is positioned to secure the necessary personal protective equipment for healthcare facilities to resume elective surgeries deemed essential."

"Given the favorable data, enhanced testing, and approval of our healthcare professionals, we will allow gyms, fitness centers, bowling alleys, body art studios, barbers, cosmetologists, hair designers, nail care artists, estheticians, their respective schools, and massage therapists to reopen their doors this Friday, April 24, 2020. Unlike other businesses, these entities have been unable to manage inventory, deal with payroll, and take care of administrative items while we shelter in place. This measure allows them to undertake baseline operations that most other businesses in the state have maintained since I issued the shelter-in-place order."

"This measure will apply statewide and will be the operational standard in all jurisdictions. This means local action cannot be taken that is more or less restrictive."

"The next point is an important one. The entities that I am reopening are not reopening for 'business as usual.' Each of these entities will be subject to specific restrictions, including adherence to Minimum Basic Operations, social distancing, and regular sanitation." "Minimum Basic Operations includes, but is not limited to, screening workers for fever and respiratory illness, enhancing workplace sanitation, wearing masks and gloves if appropriate, separating workspaces by at least six feet, teleworking where at all possible, and implementing staggered shifts."

"Subject to specific social distancing and sanitation mandates, theaters, private social clubs, and restaurant dine-in services will be allowed to reopen on Monday, April 27. We will release more information in the next few days."

"Bars, nightclubs, operators of amusement park rides, and live performance venues will remain closed. In the days ahead, we will be evaluating the data and conferring with public health officials to determine the best course of action for those establishments. "

"…The shelter in place order is still active and will expire at 11:59 PM on April 30 for most Georgians. We urge everyone to continue to follow CDC and DPH guidance by sheltering in place as often as you can. Limit your travel and limit who goes with you on errands to prevent potential exposure. If possible, wear face masks or cloth coverings when you are in public to slow the spread of coronavirus. For medically fragile and elderly Georgians, make plans to shelter in place at least through May 13 – the date Georgia's Public Health Emergency expires. …. We will release more details as we near the end of the month so medically fragile and elderly Georgians will have adequate time to prepare. I continue to call on my fellow Georgians to protect our elderly, limit your direct contact, and help them navigate the weeks ahead."

"Do what you can to help those in need. For places of worship, holding in-person services is allowed, but under Phase One guidelines, it must be done in accordance with strict social distancing protocols. I urge faith leaders to continue to help us in this effort and keep their congregations safe by heeding the advice of public health officials. Of course, online, call-in, or drive-in services remain good options for religious institutions."

"We will have tough conversations about the budget, state spending, and our priorities and values as a state. Those conversations are underway, and here's what I know: if we remain united just as we have in this fight against COVID-19, we can overcome the challenges and obstacles ahead. But if we allow politics, partisanship, elections, and egos to divide us during this important inflection point, our entire state will suffer. So, as we begin this process – this measured, deliberate step forward – let's reaffirm our commitment to each other, to the greater good, and to Georgia's future."

"I am confident that together, we will emerge victorious from this war. With your help and God's grace, we will build a safer, stronger, and more prosperous state for our families and generations to come. Thank you, and God Bless."

Soon, after Georgia, other states began to open, phase by phase. Some backing up when citizens began to congregate in the thousands at California beaches. All thoughtfully considered how and when they could try to open and resume life as a new normal.

April 9, 2020: Easter Week

Easter 2020 was the year when churches had to revert to virtual services amid the virus affecting our country. The Stay-At-Home Orders were given; or as they said, "guidelines." So, for some weeks which turned into months and a year, there were no church services. Ministers at churches recorded and showed videos of the service on the computer; special computer applications like *You Tube* and *Facebook*. So, on this Easter, Sunday, April 12th, services became familial and private as each family celebrated in their own fashion. Since mid-March that had been the new reality. Congregations remained safely at home but in communication with other church member; in most cases, through phones and computers.

Since it was allowed to check on family members, I (the author) had direct contact with my parents, aged 93 and 90, Herman and Erika Faircloth of Supply, NC and my brother and his wife, James and Rema Faircloth. "All came to my house for an Easter lunch complete with Boston Butt, greasy rice, biscuits, collards, and banana pudding; truly a southern meal. Dad led us in the Easter blessing, as usual. Just as we were finishing our meal, another family member, my niece, Nicole and her husband, David Bullard, and family, called and asked if Dad (better known as Poppa) could lead them in a prayer for their meal. We all got on a video phone so we could see each other (Face-time) and Poppa said the Easter prayer for their family. Then, my daughter, Jennifer Fisher and her family, called us, and Poppa led them in prayer for their meal. One hundred miles away but close in heart. What a wonderful Easter…with family near in our hearts even though they were miles apart and quarantined."[36]

Shortly after Easter, funding for the World Health Organization was stopped while investigations were implemented into its role in *"severely mismanaging and covering up the spread of coronavirus."*

April 16, 2020

"It is April 16th, 2020, and today may be the day that the Coronavirus Stay-at-Home Order is eased," thought many in North Carolina. Over the past month, and a bit, the President of the United States, the Governor of North Carolina, and most of the other governors, ordered residents to "stay-at-home." Of course, necessary travel to the grocery store and medical facilities, or other deemed essential services were allowed. Quick visits to other chain stores, such as Lowes and Home Depot were also allowed. The amount of business they have done in the garden centers was absolutely mind-boggling. With stay at home orders, it was the time to get the yard all ready for spring and summer and complete home projects. With the continued orders from governors on operating procedures, eventually this led to a one-way in and one-way out of the big box stores and limited numbers of folks allowed in at any one time. This, of course, applied to those who still had an income and did not worry about a lack of wages. Many were not in the position to spend any funds on frivolities.

The scary thing was that the quick and short trips to anyplace outside of your own home put you at risk of catching the virus. It was assumed that many folks could be carriers of the virus but still have no symptoms. Therefore, the recommendation was for all to wear some type of mask over their faces. At first, only those with symptoms or perhaps exposed to the virus were advised to wear masks. Most were on board with this idea to cover the nose and mouth even though not symptomatic or around anyone who had been exposed or had symptoms. Earlier, last week, *all* were advised to wear the masks.

Gloves were an added protection to avoid touching items, door knobs, gas pump handles, and anything else that another person has touched recently. Luckily, our search and rescue team had just ordered plenty of gloves prior to the initial outbreak which spread across the states. So, gloves have become my personal practice as I filled up my vehicle with gas, much like many others as word spread that this was another way the virus could spread rapidly. Although it is rarely that we need to fill up the car with gas in the past few months; we are all at home. None of us really has the desire or permission to shop at will

---

[36] Joyce Christine Judah family recollections of Easter 2020.

or drive around or visit with others. In the meantime, the price of gas dramatically dropped. They dropped considerably, due to over production by Saudi Arabia and Russia. Prices are at $1.39 per gallon here in Shallotte, North Carolina. The U. S. has stocked up their national supplies and wanted to help both of those countries by leveling the gas prices through intervention by President, Donald J. Trump. This was important to preserve the workers and companies producing the United States gas supplies and avoid the loss of those production careers. By March of 2021, prices had soared under the new President Joe Biden's administration to over $3 dollars a gallon. But that is another story.

Many were suffering from unemployment and statistics showed that it is the highest in many years as businesses stayed closed due to the states and federal government orders. Folks were split as to whether to open the economy, as it is called, since we have been basically closed down since the beginning of April and owners could not hold on much longer with no income. More testing and the ability to do contact tracing is needed to get everything back open and our leaders are trying to do it in a safe way instead of just opening everything back up and then, get a resurgence of the virus. Local health departments tried to trace all contacts with a known case to quarantine for 14 days.

In late April, the nation awaited the President to announce any national plans to re-open the economy while protestors in Michigan were lining the streets wanting everything open back up now. Other states dutifully, most often, are following the recommendations of the Centers for Disease Control and our President.

April 17th, 2020

April 17th began with the guidelines that the President and his Corona Virus Task Force had recommended with no immediate relief of all the guidelines but instead considering three main steps to getting back to normal. A disappointment for many people but a very smart, well-thought through plan, based on science statistics, and the recommendations of many business and community leaders who were consulted. A step toward normalcy was anticipated in a few months. That did not happen.

The North Carolina plan stated that maintaining social distancing will give us the best chance to manage the growing number of COVID-19 infections. Social distancing was the current practice keeping at least six feet away from the nearest person. With social distancing, it is hoped and potentially shown in the past several weeks that it does work to diminish the spread of COVID-19, lessening the strain on the medical supplies and facilities.

The U. S. was in the midst of reaching its peak and not expected to do so till mid-May. So, everyone had no choice but to still continue to follow the guidelines until further was known. They said lifting all social distancing policies soon after April 29th may lead to a situation where the hospital beds will not be available, although some think that is an over exaggeration at the least but understand the state leaders must continue to do what they feel is in the best interest of all. Most will follow the rules.

The challenge the leaders now faced was how to implement a strategy to maintain the lower levels and not provide an avenue for increased risk of infection and death. People remembering those whose families cannot visit them in the hospital as they face their final days, just elevates the angst of the general population who are even more thankful that we have the medical staff and nurses who go out of their way to comfort them. These individuals are connecting them with their families via computer face timing, and allowing families to say last words and have a final picture of their loved ones even as they take their final breaths. Tears flow from families and health care workers alike; especially when the shift is over and it is time to rest for a few hours before returning to the grueling task of caring for COVID victims.

In one hospital, the husband and wife were both stricken with the virus and above their beds were signs naming them husband and wife. This was the only situation where a family could be together at this time. This happened multiple times as the spread of the virus often infected all members of a household.

Here in Brunswick County, North Carolina, several families who came here to escape their home states where the situation was worse and who had a vacation home here, led to the entire family getting the virus, increasing the numbers in our county by 8 as of today in late April. Getting worse and being admitted to the hospital and placed on a ventilator just broke everyone's heart; whether resident or non-resident. Such a sad situation but one in which nurses understand and try to do what they can to help the patient and family as they come off the ventilators to meet their maker.

When the patient actually survives, the nurses and doctors actually dance in the hallways at saving another human being. And our hearts bleed watching those videos on television.

While the state leaders plan their strategy to open back up a state, just as each state is doing, we waited; still confined and on some version of a lockdown. We were anticipating that some states will continue requiring the wearing of facial masks when entering stores or being in crowds of more than a few people. Most plan to wear a mask for many weeks, if not longer, until this pandemic has settled down. Everyone waited on direction from state leaders, while all follow television reports daily. It almost became an addiction watching the latest on COVID. Some even became mentally affected; even suicidal in this environment.

The health departments were all trying to contain the virus in the evolving situation by monitoring specific individuals with symptoms, advising the person to isolate and quarantine for 14 days, and conducting contact tracing to identify all persons exposed to the virus from an infected individual. It was hoped that this method of containment and mitigation would prevent the spread of the disease, and even if it does not, will delay the spread providing time to prepare for peak periods which are expected to strain personnel and resources.

The mitigation, provided by the federal Task Force appointed by the President, provided guidance on personal, environmental and community measures to assist providers in risk assessment and hopefully limiting the spread of the illness. Everyone was grateful for all of those Task Force members who look tired and are working such long hours to manage this virus. It is evident on their faces that they are also feeling the strain. We all faced the strain.

May 2020

Governor Phil Murphy of New Jersey, said his state opening is dependent upon data. Some, like the Governor of California who had opened some of the beaches, were now closing them back up due to thousands who flocked there despite social distancing.

The CDC sent officials to meat packing plants to determine if they could remain open despite outbreaks of the corona virus.

Thirty million Americans were unemployed which may have a great impact for decades. This may turn out to be the worst unemployment numbers since the Great Depression.

There was still widespread hope that things would improve once states began opening back up. At this time many events were cancelled and even Fourth of July celebrations were put on hold. Most decisions were based in the numbers. But Governor Eric Holcomb, of Indiana who saw one of the largest increases in death statistics, decided to open his state back up despite a one day death toll of 1,175 people. He wanted his state to return to normal by July 4th 2020. (Nah did not happen).

Around the country, in Ohio, as of May 1st, day surgery could resume. Protestors continued to want to get their state back open while Governor DeWine gave his press conference.

In Michigan, Governor Whitmer allowed residential and commercial construction and real estate activities to resume as of May 7th. Cases in that state increased to 42,356 cases as of May 1st.

Worldwide, the world wonders if Kim Jong Uns' disappearance from any North Korea activity for the past 20 days ends the speculation that he is dead or incapacitated. He appeared in a golf cart and made his first appearance in weeks. Others wonder if this video of him riding in the golf cart is an up-to-date video or one from the past. The mystery continues, for now but it appears he is back.

———

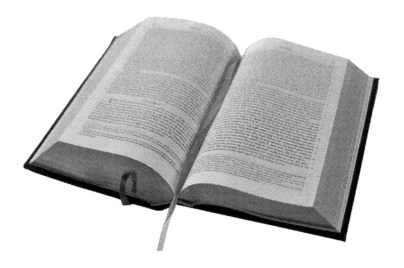

Philippians 4:13 - I can do all things through him who strengthens me.

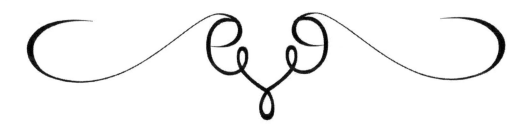

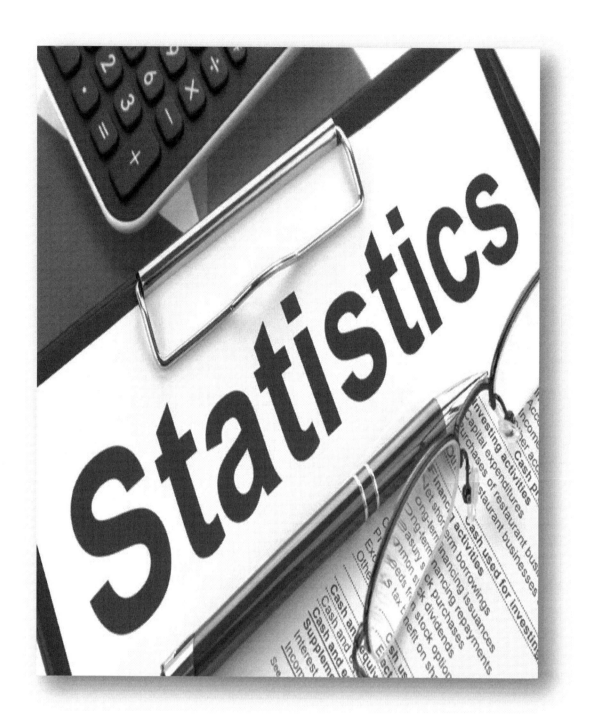

Chapter 4

Covid Statistics and News

Statistics begin to tell the story of the increasing cases in the U. S. and across the world.

Demographic characteristics of COVID-19 cases in the United States, as of April 15, 2020 *(n=465,995).*

Age groups	Cases
Less than 18	8,171
18-44	168,730
45-64	172,124
65-74	50,516
75+	
Subtotal	53,246
Unknown	13,208
Total	46,995

The cumulative total number of COVID-19 cases in the United States by report date, **January 12, 2020 to April 15, 2020**, at 4pm ET (n=632,548)

Cases of COVID-19 Reported in the U.S. by Source of Exposure

Travel-related	6,814
Close contact	14,728
Under investigation	611,006
Total cases	632,548

*On **April 14, 2020**, CDC case counts and death counts included both confirmed and probable cases and deaths. This change was made to reflect an interim COVID-19 position statement issued by the Council for State and Territorial Epidemiologists on April 5, 2020. The position statement included a case definition and made COVID-19 a nationally notifiable disease.

April 16th, 2020 - U.S. at a Glance*

Statistics according to the Center for Disease Control on April 16, 2020 showed:

Total cases: 632,548 (632,220 confirmed; 348 probable)

59

Total deaths: 31,071 (26,930 confirmed; 4,141 probable)

Jurisdictions reporting cases: 55 (50 states, District of Columbia, Guam, Puerto Rico, the Northern Mariana Islands, and the U.S. Virgin Islands).

*On April 14, 2020, CDC case counts and death counts included both confirmed and probable cases and deaths. This change was made to reflect an interim COVID-19 position statement issued by the Council for State and Territorial Epidemiologists on April 5, 2020. The position statement included a case definition and made COVID-19 a nationally notifiable disease.

State and local public health departments were now testing and publicly reporting their cases. In the event of a discrepancy between CDC cases and cases reported by state and local public health officials, data reported by states was considered the most up to date.

A confirmed case or death was defined by meeting confirmatory laboratory evidence for COVID-19. A probable case or death is defined by (i) meeting clinical criteria AND epidemiologic evidence with no confirmatory laboratory testing performed for COVID-19; or (ii) meeting presumptive laboratory evidence AND either clinical criteria OR epidemiologic evidence; or (iii) meeting vital records criteria with no confirmatory laboratory testing performed for COVID19.

According to numbers posted on April 17, 2020 by Fox News, the following statistics brought us up to date on the death rates, the saddest part of this virus. While some did not even know they had the virus and had no symptoms at all, others died within days or hours. This enhanced the general fear of the general public. **COVID was indeed deadly.**

"As of Friday morning (April 17, 2020), the novel coronavirus had infected more than 2,172,031 people across 185 countries and territories, resulting in over 146,071 deaths. In the U.S., all 50 states plus the District of Columbia had reported confirmed cases of COVID-19, tallying over 671,425 illnesses and at least 33,286 deaths".[37] This would later grow to half a million deaths in the United States by March 2021.

COVID Statistics

April 17, 2020: Case Counts[38]

>Globally: 2,196,109 cases with 149,024 deaths.
>United States: 672,303 cases with 33,898 deaths.

As an example, North Carolina statistics are described and perhaps indicative of how the virus hit various age groups and sexes.

---

[37] https://www.foxnews.com/health/coronavirus-in-us-state-by-state-breakdown. March 17, 2020.
[38] John Hopkins Data as of April 17, 2020 at 11 am.

North Carolina – April 17, 2020: 5,859 cases with 152 deaths.

429 currently hospitalized
45% male, 53% female and 2% unknown
67% of deaths were male and 33% female

Age groups

0-17	1% of cases and 0% deaths
18-24	7% of cases and 0% of deaths
25-49	38% of cases and 5% of deaths
50-64	28% of cases and 11% of deaths
65+	26% of cases and 84% of deaths

Brunswick County Residents: 36 cases with 2 deaths.
Number of Test Samples reported to the County: 1015
Pending Test Sample Results: 35
Positive Tests Results reported to county: 36
Negative Test Results reported to county: 944

Brunswick County Non-residents: 8 known cases
0 isolated at home
2 isolated at hospital
1 death
4 currently recovered
1 transferred monitoring to home residence
63 % male and 38% female
25% ages 25-49; 13% ages 50-64, and 63% over the age of 65
Death was over the age of 65

On April the 17th, 2020, California had the following statistics:

Southern California Area Statistics

Location	Cases	Deaths
Los Angeles County, California	11,391	495
Orange County, California	1,501	28
Riverside County, California	2,457	69
San Bernardino County, California	1,032	47
Ventura County, California	396	13
Total cases:	16,777	
Total deaths:		652

Sunday, April 19, 2020 White House Task Force Briefing

Millions had been tested. Tomorrow the Vice President would lead a call with the nation's governors to guide them in what they needed to do next in testing and explain how the laboratories could assist. Various labs had a tremendous capacity and could test quickly. Those could be accessed. Millions of swabs were being collected. "In the end, we will have a tremendous success," said President Trump.

The President went on to say he is "so proud of all the people who have worked so hard to handle this pandemic. We are close to finalizing a partnership to produce over 10 million swabs per month. We will use the Defense Production Act to produce more swabs. We are working with the world class team to produce over 10 million collection tubes per week."

He continued with, "Mike's team with the task force have been meeting every day and doing a great job." "Governors wanted to have total control over the opening of their states but now want to have us, the federal government, to help with testing. Testing is a local thing. We are going to get it done to the level in a short period of time as testing materials are already there."

"We will make sure everything goes well as we did with ventilators and face masks. I spoke with the President of Mexico and we will be helping them with ventilators. The number of new hospital admissions is significantly down. People have just been damaged by this scourge. We continue to see improvement in Seattle, and (other places). Nothing has happened like this since 1917. What the American people have done is incredible. They have learned a lot about washing hands, distancing and all the things we have talked about. They get it. In some places they are ready to go and other places not yet."

"One of the countries is having a big problem by not addressing this virus with restrictions. We would have had millions to die if we had not closed our borders banning people from coming in from China. It looks like we will be at about the 60 thousand mark with all the guidelines."

He continued with, "There are new guidelines for doctors and patients to be able to resume elective surgeries. As long as the rate of infection remains low, we want patients to go to their doctors and be tested, and resume preventive care. If you need a treatment in person, you should be able to get it now."

Trump said, "My administration continues to execute the massive military operations to provide beds, supplies, and equipment. We built a little more than we needed for New York and Louisiana and that is good. You have to do buildings or tents, etc. but the Army Corp of Engineers were fantastic."

"The federal government is now procuring more than 100,000 ventilators with thousands already delivered. Now New York is taking their excess ventilators and sending to Massachusetts (400). No one who needed a ventilator was denied, including in New York."

"This viral war is being fought in 184 countries around the world. Reopening our country will be tied to declining hospital admissions and testing; thanks to many other individuals and companies, labs, and agencies," said the President.

"FEMA is continuing to work to procure more gowns of the highest quality. We thank American's textile companies, who are going to produce over 5,000 gowns by the end of the month. Honeywell began producing masks in less than 5 weeks. They will produce more than 20 million masks a month. We will receive another 40 million masks in the next month. This production in addition to the 50 million already distributed. We are now approaching providing 500 million masks. In addition, we sterilize masks now. They can be sterilized up to 20 times. To put these numbers in prospective, America uses 25 million masks in a typical year," said President Trump.

"More than anything else we need to make product in the United States which is what I ran on." He then began a summary of the trade deals and dealings with China. "But with the virus, I am not happy with China. This is not a good thing. We are not in a position where we will say much yet, but all has to be taken into account as people all over the world are dying. Many countries have had their economies shattered. If we have learned something, we have learned about supply chains. A good lesson is learned."

Trump said, "Out of country supply chains do not work during rough, bad or dangerous times. To have so many products made by other countries is not good."

"Investigations are going on with the World Trade Organization and the World Health Organization." "In addition, we have launched new treatments and therapies and we have some things which are looking good. We have government agencies like NIH to slash red tape and speed development. Antiviral, antibody and immune therapy research is going well," said Trump.

Vice President Mike Pence then took the podium to talk about his Task Force and others who have represented a level of commitment which was inspiring to all. He thanked them all for their work. He said "More than 746,000 Americans have tested positive for the virus. More than 41,000 have lost their lives to the coronavirus." He expressed his sympathies to the families who were struggling.

Pence said, "Our large metro areas are seemingly past their peak. It is a tribute to the American people and the partnerships our President has forged. As we see this progress, continue to heed your local authorities. We will continue to work with governors of every state and the guidelines, and work in a way to consolidate the progress we have made, and move toward opening our country."

"Medical equipment through our Air Bridge is coming in from around the world and country," he said. Pence continued by saying, "Tomorrow we will be providing the nation's governors with information about the testing infrastructure which is available around the country, in their state, and updating them on our efforts to identify the kinds of supplies that are in those labs as the needs arise."

"This weekend we learned that we have given more than 4 million tests, and now testing more than 1 million a week. We will continue to scale that testing and urge governors to manage that testing in order to move forward into Phase One. We will continue testing people who have symptoms and test the vulnerable populations that we have identified as needed surveillance testing," he said.

Task Force member, Seema Verma, continued the briefing by talking about the testing plan to re-open our states and communities. She also talked about the nursing homes and that they are extraordinarily difficult to manage with this virus. She made the point that it is important that patients and their families have the information about what is going on in the nursing home, including reporting to the patients and families if there is a case of COVID-19 in the nursing home. She continued by "urging all states to keep nursing home patients safe."

The Nursing Homes/Assisted Living Facilities and like facilities, fared poorly in the COVID battle. Particularly in New York, many were sent to the facilities with COVID instead of remaining in hospitals as they tried to manage the numbers afflicted. Later in March of 2021 the Mayor of New York, Andrew Cuomo, would be the target of wrath for introducing more COVID by this practice leading to more deaths in facilities than might have otherwise occurred. On March 21, 2021, over 15,000 nursing home lives were remembered in Brooklyn, New York by family members. Fathers, grandfathers, mothers and grandmothers died alone; many not understanding why family was kept away amidst even minor dementia. The family members joined together on the streets of Brooklyn laying flowers at a memorial and expressed their sadness at not being able to be with family when they were so ill and died. Some members voiced that they wished it had been handled differently especially when they knew for weeks that their loved one was heading toward death. It was hard not to be with family to support, hold and love them in the facility.

As in all briefings, then the floor was open to reporters for questions, seated at least six feet apart for social distancing. Questions ranged from subjects about protesting people wanting to hasten the opening of states, aid to IRAN, which governors had gone too far in the restrictions, when the deal will be done for more money on small business loans (adding more funds to take care of small businesses, negotiating with the democrats), and many other questions with most briefings lasting upwards to two and a half hours.

In the meantime, around the globe some countries announced that they would issue a digital immunity card to those who have recovered from COVID. They were supposed to help identify persons who did not pose a health risk to others. This practice by Chili did not seem to catch on with the rest of the world but documentation of immunization was to become common practice in the U. S. when immunizations were given in early 2021.

While the pandemic continued around the world, the entire global population was eager to get back to the "new normal." Exactly what the new normal will be was of yet unknown. People all over the world locked down to try to get control of the viral infections. Statistics documenting cases and deaths rose.

In the United States… alphabetically:

	Cases Reported April 23, 2020	Cases Reported June 6, 2021	
Alabama	4,241	546,249	
Alaska	293	67,648	
American Samoa	0	N/A	
Arizona	3,962	883,314	
Arkansas	1,583	342,345	
California	24,424	3,688,893	
Colorado	8,280	546,500	
Connecticut	14,755	347,891	
Delaware	2,014	109,070	
Washington D.C.	2,197	49,068	
Florida	21,865	2,286,332	
Georgia	15.409	1,125,854	
Guam	135	8,204	
Hawaii	517	35,283	
Idaho	1,587	192,854	
Illinois	24,593	1,384,903	
Indiana	8,955	746,554	
Iowa	1,995	371,956	
Kansas	1,494	314,855	
Kentucky	2,291	460,412	
Louisiana	21,951	472,981	
Maine	770	68,232	
Marshall Islands	0	4	
Maryland	10,784	460,575	
Massachusetts	29,918	707,940	

	Cases Reported April 23, 2020	Cases Reported June 6, 2021	
Michigan	28,059	994,935	
Micronesia	0	0	
Minnesota	1,862	602,428	
Mississippi	3,624	318,189	
Missouri	4,895	602,019	
Montana	415	112,260	
Nebraska	952	223,558	
Nevada	3,211	325,392	
New Hampshire	1,139	98,877	
New Jersey	71,030	1,017,695	
New Mexico	1,484	203,472	
New York	211,550	1,152,913	
			"Queens's hospital has body bags all over the floor of the hospital." D. J. Trump.
North Carolina	5,123	1,004,669	
North Dakota	365	110,199	
Northern Marianas	13	183	
Ohio	7,791	1,104,380	
Oklahoma	2,263	453,796	
Oregon	1,663	202,995	
Palau	0	4	
Pennsylvania	26,490	1,205,290	
Puerto Rico	974	139,004	
Rhode Island	3,529	151,992	

	Cases Reported April 23, 2020	Cases Reported June 76 2021	
South Carolina	3,656	594,264	
South Dakota	1,168	124,261	
Tennessee	5836	863,840	
Texas	15,492	2,952,601	
Utah	2,637	407,419	
Vermont	759	24,252	
Virgin Islands	51	3,591	
Virginia	6,889	676,741	
	It was widely reported that the Governor of Virginia wanted to take away guns in his state. Gun sales rose and ammunition became scarce.	It remains scarce as of the end of March 2021 and when available, prices are often $60 for a box of 50, 9 mm bullets versus the previous costs, rising by upwards to 400% per box.	This continues to be an issue across the nation and continues in June of 2021.
Washington	10,783	440,057	
West Virginia	718	162,232	
Wisconsin	3,721	675,150	
Wyoming	393	60,628	

Worldwide Statistics for Comparisons	Confirmed Cases April 23, 2020	Confirmed Cases June 6, 2021	Deaths June 6, 2021
	833,627	173,005,553	3,727,605
	Today + 285		
	Deaths, 42,302 Today +38		
US Data on April 27, 2020 Over 55,563 had died.	In the United States, over 979,077 cases have been diagnosed as of April 27, 2020.	A of April 27th, 2020, the top three states with the highest statistics are New York, Massachusetts, and New Jersey.	
United States and Territories Statistics in order of the Highest Confirmed Cases on April 23, 2020	Cases Apr 23, 2020	Deaths April 23, 2020	Deaths June 6, 2021
New York State	257,216	15,063	19,818
New Jersey	95,,865	5,063	26,273
Massachusetts	42,,944	2182	17,907
California	37,629	1,430	62,242
Pennsylvania	35684	1,622	27,349
Illinois	35,,107	1,565	25,314
Michigan	33,966	2,813	20,588
Florida	28,576	927	36,973
Louisiana	25,258	1,473	10,615
Connecticut	22,469	1,544	8,246
Georgia	21,102	846	20,986
Texas	21,069	543	50,621
Maryland	14,775	631	9,644
Ohio	14,117	610	19,980
Washington	12,494	692	5,836
Indiana	12,438	661	13,685
Colorado	10,878	508	6,613
Virginia	10,878	349	11,236

United States and Territories Statistics in order of the Highest Confirmed Cases on April 23, 2020	Cases Apr 23, 2020	Deaths April 23, 2020	Deaths June 6, 2021
Tennessee	7,842	166	12,476
North Carolina	7,220	242	13,151
Missouri	6,137	208	9,140
Rhode Island	5,841	181	2,717
Alabama	5,610	201	11,215
Arizona	5,469	229	17,698
Mississippi	4,894	193	7,325
Wisconsin	4,845	246	7,954
South Carolina	4,761	140	9,770
Nevada	4,081	172	5,600
Iowa	3,748	90	6,068
Utah	3,445	34	2,311
Kentucky	3,373	185	7,091
Delaware	3,200	89	1,677
Oklahoma	2,894	170	7,324
Minnesota	2,721	179	7,554
Arkansas	2,3692	44	5,846
Kansas	2,211	110	5,084
New Mexico	2,210	71	4,280
Oregon	2,059	78	2,691
South Dakota	1,858	9	2,022
Idaho	1,802	54	2,105
Nebraska	1,802	38	2,249
New Hampshire	1,588	48	1,355
West Virginia	963	29	2,813
Maine	907	39	839
Vermont	823	40	256
North Dakota	679	14	1,516
Hawaii	592	12	499
Montana	439	14	1,632
Alaska	335	9	362
Wyoming	326	6	720
Puerto Rico			2,518
District of Columbia			1,136
Micronesia	0	0	0

United States and Territories Statistics in order of the Highest Confirmed Cases on April 23, 2020	Cases Apr 23, 2020	Deaths April 23, 2020	Deaths June 6, 2021
Guam			139
Virgin Islands			28
Mariana Islands			2
Palau			0
Republic of Marshall Islands			0
Total		**51,876**	**594,3381**

++Sources of all US data from the Center for Disease Control.

Situation by World Health Organization Region++

Confirmed Cases on June 6, 2021

Americas - 68,533,720

Europe – 54,665,868

South-East Asia - 32,772,064

Eastern Mediterranean - 10,302,176

Africa - 3,573,298

Western Pacific - 3,157,663

++Source: World Health Organization, June 6, 2021.

The News across the U. S. – Watching the Headlines late April 2020

Many aspects of the virus were being exposed in news articles across the world. So many aspects of the virus were being written about. A sampling of those articles included:

Drones Detecting Wealthy Social Distancing Violators: Draganfly Inc. announced on April 21, 2020, the first-ever series of U.S. 'pandemic drone' test flights in Westport, Connecticut, considered a COVID-19 'hotspot', to identify social distancing and detect symptoms presented by the...

Apr 22: **Saliva More Sensitive Than Swabs for SARS-CoV2 Tests:** A non-peer-reviewed study published on April 22, 2020, finds saliva is a viable and more sensitive alternative to nasopharyngeal swabs and could enable at-home self-administered sample collection for accurate large-scale SARS-CoV-2...

Apr 22: United Kingdom Deaths 42,302   Today: +38

Apr 22: **Cats Are Not Spreading Coronavirus:** According to Dr. Anthony Fauci's response during a TV press conference on April 22, 2020, pets such as common cats, are not carriers of the SARS-CoV-2 coronavirus. Dr. Fauci, a director with the... (However, later, two tigers in the zoo contracted it and it is said to have been diagnosed in other animals as well.)

Apr 22: RT-PCR **Test Results Can Mislead Coronavirus Diagnosis:** A new study reported the extended existence of SARS-CoV-2 coronavirus in some asymptomatic patients can reach 26 days. And, asymptomatic SARS-CoV-2 carriers are important potential infection sources of COVID-19 disease and may have...

Apr 22: **California Actually Confirmed Initial COVID-19 Fatalities:** Santa Clara County, California, health officials announced on April 21, 2020, that at least 2 fatalities during February are now attributed to COVID-19 disease. Both fatalities in Santa Clara County had...

Apr 22: **Air Sensor May Detect SARS-CoV-2:** A team of researchers from Empa, ETH Zurich, and Zurich University Hospital announced April 21, 2020, that they succeeded in developing a novel sensor for detecting the SARS-CoV-2 coronavirus. This means, in the...

Coronavirus News on April 23, 2020

Apr 23: **Coronavirus Today** www.coronavirustoday.com

Coronavirus Today publishes vaccine news patients can trust to make informed immunization decisions in partnership with doctors, nurses, and pharmacists

Apr 23: China denies coronavirus originated from Wuhan lab.

Apr 23: Coronavirus: Latest News and Updates on the COVID-19 Outbreak ... www.dailymail.co.uk/news/coronavirus coronavirus. Australia goes into voluntary administration putting 15,000 jobs at risk - but it will keep operating while it restructures 21...

More headlines that Appeared in the Next Few Weeks...

FDA Authorizes First Test for Patient At-Home Sample Collection

Laboratory Corporation of America COVID-19 RT-PCR Test permits self-collected samples to be tested for SARS-CoV-2 coronavirus

CMS Issues Recommendations to Re-Open Healthcare Systems

Guidelines for Opening Up America Again with a relatively low and stable incidence of COVID-19 cases

Visualizing Vaccine Development through Antibody Mapping

CR3022 cross-reacts with the novel coronavirus, although the antibody doesn't bind tightly enough to neutralize it from infecting cells

COVID-19 Vaccine & Treatment Development Accelerated from Public-Private Partnerships

Accelerating COVID-19 Therapeutic Interventions and Vaccines (ACTIV) empowers industry collaborations

Plasma Needed from Recovered COVID-19 Patients

FDA encourages coronavirus recovered patients to donate plasma to expedite therapy development

Ophthalmologist could be infected with SARS-CoV-2 when treating patients

COVID-19 Antibody Testing Free with Private Insurance

CMS removes financial barriers to receive COVID-19 tests and health services

Make a Difference during the Coronavirus Pandemic

Slow the spread of the SARS-CoV-2 coronavirus by taking action

Largest COVID-19 Antibodies Study Launches

Helping Quantify Coronavirus Outbreak from Your Home

SARS-CoV-2 infections can be detected by analyzing blood for antibodies

Tech Titans Empower Contact Tracing's Digital Synchronization

Google and Apple deploy Bluetooth Low Energy tech for contact tracing platform

Only 19% of Americans Are Self-Isolating

COVID-19 disease pandemic-initiated lifestyle changes in the USA

Serological Tests Can Detect COVID-19 Disease

FDA issued policy enabling early access to certain serological tests

Coronavirus Aerosolized Through Talking

SARS-CoV-2 viral particles cause COVID-19 disease

Swiss Fast-Tracking Hydroxychloroquine Treatments for Hospitalized COVID-19 Patients

6-Steps to Crush the COVID-19 Curve

Blood Cancer Patients Have Options for Coronavirus Treatment

Exquisitely Seeing How Corona viruses Attach to Human Cells

New Blood Donor Policies from the FDA

Enforced Social-Distancing Produces Positive Results

Diarrhea Often Present in Mild COVID-19 Disease

New Study to Eliminate Mechanical Ventilation of COVID-19 Patients

Beware of fraudulent claims of COVID-19 medicine,

No Approved Coronavirus Vaccines or Medicines Available, Yet

Italy's Coronavirus Version is a Slow-Mutating-Pathogen

Loss of Smell Can Indicate Coronavirus Infection

Mandatory Testing Can Halt Coronavirus Outbreak

Pregnant Women Advised to Avoid Suspected or COVID-19 Disease Patients

Nursing Regulations Waived to Meet COVID-19 Outbreak Needs

Blood Type A People Need to be More Vigilant

12% of Assessed Children in China Found Infected with Coronavirus

Advanced COVID-19 Treatments Can Save Lives

Coronavirus Lives on Surfaces for Days

Largest COVID-19 Antibodies Study Launches

Tech Titans Empower Contact Tracing's Digital Synchronization

FDA Authorizes First Test for Patient At-Home Sample Collection

Laboratory Corporation of America COVID-19 RT-PCR Test permits self-collected samples to be tested for SARS-CoV-2 coronavirus

CMS Issues Recommendations to Re-Open Healthcare System**s**

Guidelines for Opening-Up America Again with a relatively low and stable incidence of COVID-19 cases

FDA Coronavirus Treatment Acceleration Program moves new treatments to patients as soon as possible

Coronavirus at meat packing plants worse than first thought, USA TODAY investigation finds.

Coronavirus: Can I get a home testing kit and what is an antibody test?

How to get coronavirus-related alerts on your phone

Las Vegas Sands (LVS) Q1 Earnings Beat, Fall Y/Y on Coronavirus

The company has suspended its quarterly dividend program citing the coronavirus-induced crisis....

NBC Universal launches ads to help retailers hurt by coronavirus

U.S. TV networks are poised to lose as much as $12 billion in ad revenue in the first half of......

Reporters waited for the latest Presidential comments (From President Trump) and direction. Monitoring Fox News, his remarks for today included (with supporting presentation by Dr. Birx):

-Outbreaks in Brazil, unfortunately, are making us look at travel from Brazil. And other countries where we have a lot of product coming in from Latin America.

-Outbreaks in Florida are attributed more to travel from New York than Latin America or South America, according to Florida Governor Ron Desantis. Next steps for Florida will be announced tomorrow.

-The President says, "We have a large overcapacity of ventilators and will be sending many overseas. More than ten thousand are in the federal stockpile."

-Testing is going very well.

-Food Supply Chain: We are working with Tyson and will sign an executive order today and that will solve any liability problems. We have plenty of supply. With processing plants closed down, there is a legal roadblock. We are working on that.

-Our early bans of travel into our country from China and other countries were badly criticized when we did those, but everyone now knows and sees it was a good thing. By doing this, we saved many thousands of lives.

-I think the 4th quarter is going to be very strong. 3rd quarter is a transition quarter. And next year will be an unbelievably strong year.

The Democrats did not want to come back to Washington to vote on bills and this angered President Trump. He believed they should all come back and work on this together.

President Trump looked very tired and worn on television. It was reported he only slept a few hours each night. Patriots prayed for him and asked that "God give him the wisdom to continue guiding our country toward some type of normalcy in the near future."

Global Statistics

Globally, 3,017,806 cases of COVID have been diagnosed with 209,661 deaths. (April 27, 2020). Statistics can be found at: Coronavirus COVID-19 Global Cases by the Center for systems Science and Engineering (CSSE) at John Hopkins University (JHU).

Tracking Death

	Global	US	NC	Brunswick County, NC	
4/24/20	194,456	50,373	269	2
4/27/20	209,661	55,563	306	4
4/30/20	228,600	61,000	378	4

By April 30th, 2020, the White House "Slow the Spread" guidelines were put into place. This was a part of a nationwide effort to slow the spread of COVID-19 through the implementation of social distancing at all levels of society.

Medications

On **April 30th**, reports from the studies, evaluating over 800 virus patients, had shown it was successful in limiting the amount of time a person suffered from the symptoms, ending the symptoms in a minimum of four days less than the patient who has not received the drug. Dr. Anthony Fauci announced he is optimistic about this drug being used in the treatment of COVID.[39] He said, "Preliminary data analysis from an international COVID-19 drug trial "shows that *remdesivir* has a clear-cut, significant, positive effect in diminishing the time to recovery," Fauci told reporters at the White House Wednesday."

"This development is "really quite important for a number of reasons," Fauci said, calling the data "highly significant." He said that "the recovery time was reduced from 15 days to 11 days in the drug trial, which involved over 1,000 hospitalized patients in the U.S., Germany, Denmark, Spain, Greece and other countries, and was, he said, "the first truly high-powered, randomized, placebo-controlled" trial for a coronavirus treatment." Research into developing a vaccine continued.

News across the Nation

The news across the nation was filled with articles and new information about the Coronavirus and its effects on people across the globe. It would be literally impossible to do justice to each and every aspect of the virus. So, in the interest of a broad view of the news bombarding us during 2020, headlines are listed below to give the reader a perspective and sampling of the news. It was way too much to digest and sometimes nearly everyone had to turn off the television, put the papers down, turn off the radios and just go outside for some sunshine and yard work to relieve the stress. For others, this was a glimpse into our lives.

By March of 2021, there have been more than 842,000 coronavirus death cases in the United States, according to the Johns Hopkins University tally.[40]

States rushing to reopen are likely making a deadly error, coronavirus models and experts warn.[41]

As several states — including South Carolina, Tennessee and Florida — rush to reopen businesses, the sudden relaxation of restrictions will supply new targets for the ...[42]

People were asking the following questions…

How to make your own mask for virus protection?

What is Paracetamol? (Acetaminophen, over the counter pain reliever)

How can you track a stimulus check? (Checks nearly everyone in the nation received from the government to help defray living expenses. The first check was $600 per adult paid in December 2020/Jan 2021. Subsequent checks of $1200

---

[39] Fauci optimistic about remdesivir as treatment for COVID-19. CBS News. April 30, 2020.
[40] Washington Post. April 22, 2020.
[41] IBID.
[42] Yahoo News. April 23, 2020.

were sent to citizens later in the spring and recently, March 2021, promises to send citizens $1400 each. It is unknown at this time if additional checks will be issued to help US citizens meet the demands of unemployment and the loss of businesses, loss of jobs, etc. as a result of the pandemic.)

How do you sanitize the N95 mask?

Where can I stream online concerts?

When are we going back to work?

Does anyone understand the economic hardship on us?

Why are protestors demanding the reopening of the economy when it is still dangerous?

Will the schools be reopened anytime soon?

When do the hair and nail salons open?

How can I pay the mortgage if I am not allowed to work?

Why can some stores open and others are closed?

And hundreds of other questions echoed the uncertainty of the day…. to cope with this pandemic and the altered way of living that resulted.

Food boxes were distributed to those in need. Many senior centers or other local government offices distributed limited numbers of boxes containing a gallon of milk, some cheese, yogurt, five pounds of potatoes, a bag of fresh carrots, and some type of meat. Sometimes it was a pack of sausages, or hotdogs, or chicken legs, or some other type of bagged meat called chicken taco filling but looking more like an undetermined red clump. You might also get a couple of onions and some oranges thrown in. A cardboard box of food to help the poor, coupled with a long line of cars scheduled to pick it up on Friday mornings; or other days depending upon distribution center. Swallowing your pride, many lined up to get this little bit of help. Some were disappointed when too many signed up and they were not given a box. A slow drive back home without your taters. Ask and you could get a box, but the limited supply was apparent. This ended about June 2021 in North Carolina….with an unknown status in other states.

———

Global efforts by **April 2020** were focused on lessening the spread and impact of this virus. The federal government worked closely with state, local, tribal, and territorial partners, as well as public health partners, to respond to this public health threat. CDC responded to a pandemic of respiratory disease spreading from person-to-person caused by a novel (new) coronavirus and named "coronavirus disease 2019." They described the situation as posing a serious public health risk.

Even the person who tried to limit personal exposure to news reports found themselves with a headache just trying to process all the information being provided in the media. It was impossible to avoid being bombarded daily and with one eye closed, everyone wanted to know the latest information and what the future held. But no one really knew.

In the United States, there were 54,299 newly reported COVID-19 cases and 973 newly reported COVID-19 deaths on **Mar 17, 2021**. [43]

State level Stats in the following chart show the cases on **March 17th, 2021** and trends according to the last 14 days.[44]

	Total Cases	Total Deaths	Mortality Rate
California [#1]	3,634,807 9.2% pop	57,200 0.1% pop	1.6%
Texas [#2]	2,745,817 9.5% pop	47,025 0.2% pop	1.7%
Florida [#3]	1,994,117 9.3% pop	32,598 0.2% pop	1.6%
New York [#4]	1,767,290 9.1% pop	49,262 0.3% pop	2.8%
Illinois [#5]	1,215,992 9.6% pop	23,287 0.2% pop	1.9%
Georgia [#6]	1,040,817 9.8% pop	18,420 0.2% pop	1.8%
Ohio [#7]	995,785 8.5% pop	17,991 0.2% pop	1.8%

---

[43] IBID.
[44]Data Sources: John Hopkins CSSE, CDC Testing Report; https://COVIDusa.net/
References: https://www.aha.org/statistics/fast-facts-us-hospitals
http://www.centerforhealthsecurity.org/cbn/2020/cbnreport-02272020.html
https://www.statnews.com/2020/03/10/simple-math-alarming-answers-COVID-19/
https://www.cdc.gov/flu/about/burden/index.html
https://COVIDactnow.org/

	Total Cases	Total Deaths	Mortality Rate
Pennsylvania [8]	979,638 7.7% pop	24,722 0.2% pop	2.5%
North Carolina [9]	891,314 8.5% pop	11,783 0.1% pop	1.3%
New Jersey [10]	853,188 9.6% pop	24,076 0.3% pop	2.8%
Arizona [11]	834,607 11.5% pop	16,645 0.2% pop	2%
Tennessee [12]	796,624 11.7% pop	11,681 0.2% pop	1.5%
Michigan [13]	683,398 6.8% pop	16,843 0.2% pop	2.5%
Indiana [14]	675,388 10% pop	12,907 0.2% pop	1.9%
Wisconsin [15]	627,743 10.8% pop	7,208 0.1% pop	1.1%
Massachusetts [16]	608,318 8.8% pop	16,759 0.2% pop	2.8%
Virginia [17]	600,550 7% pop	10,182 0.1% pop	1.7%
Missouri [18]	574,015 9.4% pop	8,709 0.1% pop	1.5%
South Carolina [19]	537,498 10.4% pop	8,938 0.2% pop	1.7%
Alabama [20]	510,048 10.4% pop	10,391 0.2% pop	2%
Minnesota [21]	501,458 8.9% pop	6,830 0.1% pop	1.4%
Colorado [22]	446,580	6,060	1.4%

	Total Cases	Total Deaths	Mortality Rate
	7.8% pop	0.1% pop	
Louisiana [23]	439,543 9.5% pop	9,974 0.2% pop	2.3%
Oklahoma [24]	432,793 10.9% pop	4,788 0.1% pop	1.1%
Kentucky [25]	419,149 9.4% pop	5,504 0.1% pop	1.3%
Maryland [26]	396,746 6.6% pop	8,113 0.1% pop	2%
Utah [27]	380,340 11.9% pop	2,041 0.1% pop	0.5%
Iowa [28]	363,433 11.5% pop	5,672 0.2% pop	1.6%
Washington [29]	352,907 4.6% pop	5,168 0.1% pop	1.5%
Arkansas [30]			
Mississippi [31]	301,924 10.1% pop	6,938 0.2% pop	2.3%
Kansas [32]	301,085 10.3% pop	4,793 0.2% pop	1.6%
Nevada [33]	300,415 9.8% pop	5,157 0.2% pop	1.7%
Connecticut [34]	295,484 8.3% pop	7,822 0.2% pop	2.6%
Nebraska [35]	205,539 10.6% pop	2,133 0.1% pop	1%
New Mexico [36]	189,158 9% pop	3,877 0.2% pop	2%

	Total Cases	Total Deaths	Mortality Rate
Idaho [#37]	176,802 9.9% pop	1,938 0.1% pop	1.1%
Oregon [#38]	160,622 3.8% pop	2,353 0.1% pop	1.5%
West Virginia [#39]	136,716 7.6% pop	2,570 0.1% pop	1.9%
Rhode Island [#40]	132,616 12.5% pop	2,594 0.2% pop	2%
South Dakota [#41]	115,203 13% pop	1,919 0.2% pop	1.7%
Puerto Rico [#42]	103,679 3.2% pop	2,089 0.1% pop	2%
Montana [#43]	102,616 9.6% pop	1,406 0.1% pop	1.4%
North Dakota [#44]	101,403 13.3% pop	1,490 0.2% pop	1.5%
Delaware [#45]	91,425 9.4% pop	1,517 0.2% pop	1.7%
New Hampshire [#46]	79,702 5.9% pop	1,207 0.1% pop	1.5%
Alaska [#47]	61,019 8.3% pop	310 0.04% pop	0.5%
Wyoming [#48]	55,479 9.6% pop	693 0.1% pop	1.2%
Maine [#49]	48,071 3.6% pop	728 0.1% pop	1.5%
District of Columbia [#50]	42,892 6.1% pop	1,046 0.1% pop	2.4%
Hawaii [#51]	28,795	450	1.6%

	Total Cases	Total Deaths	Mortality Rate
	2% pop	0.03% pop	
Vermont [#52]	17,247 2.8% pop	217 0.03% pop	1.3%
Guam [#53]	7,780 4.7% pop	134 0.1% pop	1.7%
Virgin Islands [#54]	2,767 2.7% pop	25 0.02% pop	0.9%
Northern Mariana Islands [#55]	157 0.3% pop	19 0.03% pop	12.1%

———

The Latest National Headlines from CNN in June of 2021 [45]

- The CDC's Covid-19 vaccination card, annotated
- A lag in Covid-19 vaccinations among adolescents could delay US return to normalcy, experts warn
- Uganda reimposes Covid-19 restrictions as cases surge in second wave
- Classified report with early support for lab leak theory reemerges as focal point for lawmakers digging into Covid-19 origins
- Travel to Singapore during Covid-19: What you need to know before you go
- Hundreds of former leaders urge G7 to vaccinate poor against Covid-19
- Covid-19 cases fall, but unvaccinated children are a 'vulnerable host' for coronavirus, doctor says
- In rural Georgia, a door-to-door push to get neighbors vaccinated against Covid-19
- Golfer Jon Rahm forced to withdraw from Memorial Tournament after positive Covid-19 test

---

[45] CNN News. https://www.cnn.com/specials/world/coronavirus-outbreak-intl-hnk. June 7, 2021.

- Some US hospitals mark first time being Covid-free. Others still see surge of patients

- Vietnam sees Covid-19 surge amid potentially 'new variant'

- How a vaccination experiment known as 'Project S' transformed one small Brazilian city

- Covid-19 variant identified in India may increase risk of hospitalization, UK officials say

- Mixing coronavirus vaccine brands is OK, Canada says

  These people want to get back to work but can't -- and fear losing $300-a-week benefits will spell financial disaster

- Are unemployment benefits causing working shortages? Here's what we know.

- Fed official: Getting women back to work is about 'our economic potential as a nation'

- A lot of people are waiting for porta potties -- and not just folks who need to go

- Why some companies want everyone back in the office

- Covid-19 cases are falling, but experts say kids should still get a vaccine when they can. Here's why

- Vaccinated children can go mask-free at summer camp, says CDC

- Ohio teen wins full ride for college in vaccine giveaway

- NYC and Los Angeles schools will return to in-person classes five days a week in the fall

- What the new CDC mask guidance means for kids under 12

- Poll: Two-thirds of Americans say life is at least somewhat back to pre-pandemic normal

- Is the handshake back? How we're greeting each other as the world reopens

- The whitewashing of Arab Americans impacted by Covid-19 is a catastrophic public health issue, experts say

- Don't just go back to 'normal.' Post-pandemic life can be much better than that

  Hundreds of former leaders urge G7 to vaccinate poor against Covid-19

- Classified report with early support for lab leak theory reemerges as focal point for lawmakers digging into Covid-19 origins

- Caught in crosshairs, Fauci calls GOP descriptions of his emails 'profoundly misleading'

- Biden administration announces plan to share first 25 million Covid-19 doses abroad

- $6 trillion stimulus: Here's who got relief money so far

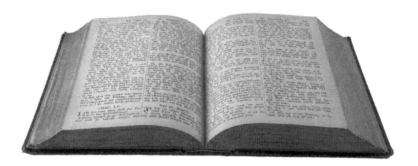

Luke 17:5 - The apostles said to the Lord, "Increase our faith!

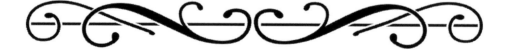

Chapter 5

The Sickness and Healthcare Providers

Dealing with the Virus

The most difficult part was *having the virus*. Individuals, famous, rich, poor, old and young were stricken and forced to deal with the virus. Some individuals shared their plight readily; others hid their illness for fear of being targeted as a *COVID-19 patient*. People were afraid.

President Trump shared that a friend of his called him one day to let him know that he had tested positive and was on his way to the hospital. The next day he was in a coma. Within short order, this gentleman, a close friend of the President, was dead. It made it real.

The risk from COVID-19 to Americans was broken down into risk of exposure versus risk of serious illness and death.

Risk of Exposure

Cases of COVID-19 and instances of community spread were reported in all states.

*People in places where ongoing community spread of the virus caused COVID-19 were at elevated risk of exposure, with the level of risk dependent on the location.

*Healthcare workers caring for patients with COVID-19 were at elevated risk of exposure.

*Close contacts of persons with COVID-19 also put one at an elevated risk of exposure.

*Travelers returning from affected international locations where community spread was occurring were at elevated risk of exposure, with level of risk dependent on where they traveled.

*People who live in a nursing home or long-term care facility, and

*People of all ages with underlying medical conditions.

The CDC developed guidance to help in the risk assessment and management of people with potential community-related exposures to COVID-19. They established three levels of risk.

Three Levels of Risk

The following three levels identified the risk of contracting the virus:

0 / No Risk: Briefly walking by a person who tested positive for the virus and not experiencing any symptoms.

1/Low Risk: Being in the same room as a person who tested positive who had symptoms and you were within six feet.

2/Medium Risk: Sustained close contact of 10 minutes or more within a six feet distance while they had symptoms.

3/High Risk: Close household contact with a person who tested positive.

Travelers

American citizens, lawful permanent residents, and their families who had been in one of the countries with travel restrictions for entering the U.S. in the past 14 days, were allowed to enter the United States but they were redirected to one of 13 airports. They were assessed and some were recommended to quarantine for 14 days all in an attempt to manage the read of the virus.

If returning from one of these target countries, you were asked to stay home and monitor your own health. All other international travelers were told to follow CDC instructions during this time. "Your cooperation is integral to the ongoing public health response to try to slow the spread of this virus," noted the CDC. By May of 2021, travel was again halted from India as their Covid numbers rose out of control with medical facilities unable to handle them, having a lack of oxygen. The second-wave had hit.

Healthcare Providers

The CDC went on to direct, "If you are a healthcare provider, use your judgment to determine if a patient has signs and symptoms compatible with COVID-19 and whether the patient should be tested." CDC's Criteria to Guide Evaluation and Laboratory Testing for COVID-19 provided priorities for testing patients with suspected COVID-19 infection. It appeared to be selective and unless an individual had multiple symptoms, it *few* were able to get a test. This changed later in the year when *most* were tested and statistics rose much higher showing how many people were indeed infected. One had to wonder how many were actually infected but did not seek testing or were turned away from accessing a test earlier in the year. Some of those people went on to infect others, perhaps unknowingly. And of course, there were those who had no symptoms but did indeed have the virus and spread it to others.

Medical Workers

Nurses were under extreme pressure in the hardest hit areas of the country. In all areas, the COVID-19 virus had all medical workers on edge, diagnosing and caring for patients.

Hospice Nurse, Wendy Long, of Southport, NC, described her experience. "From the perspective of a Hospice Nurse, things are somewhat different. In the beginning of the pandemic, people were trying to get their loved ones placed in a nursing home because they felt they would not be able to care for them." However, nursing homes were soon locked down after a wide outbreak in a home in Seattle, Washington, early in the pandemic.

Ms. Long continued, "Then, some people would not let the nurses come to their house. As a Hospice Nurse, I have been monitoring my temperature and sanitizing every time I turn around. I am lucky I can still do visits." "I have gone to four deaths in one weekend when no one else would go, because of the fear of the virus. Our patients have a terminal illness; not necessarily COVID. The funeral homes are reluctant to take the bodies also; until I reassure them our patients have had no symptoms of COVID for two weeks before they passed away. It is a new frontier and no one knows quite how to navigate it. We are making a plan as we go along."

Iris Lawes described her experiences as the wife of a medical student. "My husband and I are active, healthy, and in our late twenties. On paper, we were not what were considered 'high risk' for COVID-19. In this way, we experience this crisis in a different way than so many in this world. We also, though, loved our parents and grandparents. We are aunts and uncles to our baby nephew. And we are profoundly concerned for our country. Overall, we are simply worried for those we love." She went on to say, "In a society that so often has motivated business and progress, we find ourselves today being asked to do only one thing---absolutely nothing. Nothing but stay within the confines of our home, and find some joy out of Zoom meetings and Zoom dinners. As an accountant making her way through tax season, and a medical student navigating classes remotely, we find the dynamics of our jobs adjust to align even further with available technology."

"It is an odd place for my husband—to be so close to graduating but not yet certified to practice medicine. In a time that needs health care professionals more than ever, he is doing the best thing for everyone—to learn the most he can as fast as he can. His classes have gone virtual and although he is not on physical rotations, he still studies the topics he would be otherwise. I am so proud of him and all that he is doing. The work he is completing now will ready him to treat our country, and to do it well," Lawes stated.

She went on to say, "Outside of staying diligent with our work, we have to stay diligent in our faith. We find solace in our faith. My Bible study has continued as usual, just from the comfort of our respective living rooms. We find ourselves praying more earnestly and asking more questions about the plan that is in store. What we have found is that through all of this is the undeniable fact that people are inherently good.! People are staying home not just to help themselves, but to care for complete strangers around them. Grocery workers show up to underpaid jobs so that people can have food on the table. Nurses are caring for patients as though they are family of their own."

Lawes said, "Overall, we are thankful for each other and for our families. We are finding ways to keep busy and to keep hopeful. We are focusing on the Lord and on the good in His creation. We are grateful for our health and for those who help sustain it."

Nurses in hospitals hit with high numbers of COVID patients, were helping them to stay in touch with their families through technology, Facebook, phone and computer screens. No family was allowed into the hospitals in order to attempt to curb the spread of the virus. That was a terrorizing thing for those with dying family members inside.

Like-wise in the nursing homes, families visited by communicating through the windows with visitors staying outside the building.

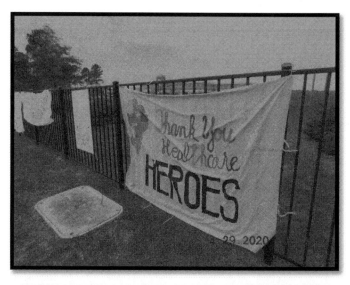

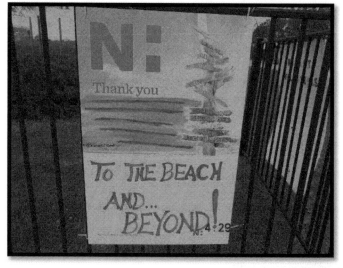

Figure 17 Banners in front of Novant Hospital, Brunswick County, NC.

The towns' people showed their support and appreciation to the medical workers by sending food and other gifts to show their appreciation. They recognized all the assistance that the medical workers provided in treating patients and putting their own lives on the line. There were even news reports of medical workers who had taken their own lives. The stress level was so high they lost their spirit to continue. Most of those medical workers, along with many other essential workers, continued to provide their services.

On April 29th, supporters posted banners in the front of the local hospital, the Novant Hospital in Supply, North Carolina. It was only a small token of the appreciation by the community and was repeated throughout the nation.

Parking lots remained empty on the front of the hospital and were blocked with construction barrels, directing patients to the emergency room entrance on the back of the hospital. Like most doctors' offices, patients were being screened first and then directed to the appropriate place for services. Often, this was done in a tent outside of the actual doctors building; in the parking lot.

Surgical centers both within hospitals and day surgery centers were beginning to open and accept patients for non-essential surgeries. This happened partly for the needed income they had lost when non-essential surgeries were halted by The White House Coronavirus Task Force guidelines. Even within hospitals and other medical facilities, many personnel were furloughed when services were cut, even though the number of patients increased with corona. In addition, many patients just stayed home rather than seek medical care from doctors or hospitals and emergency rooms, afraid of contracting the virus.

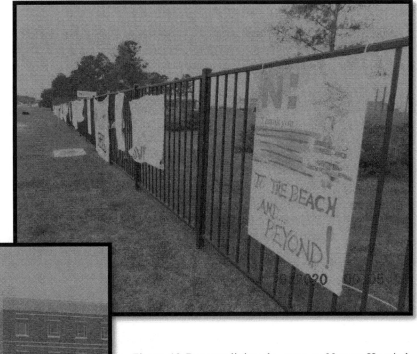

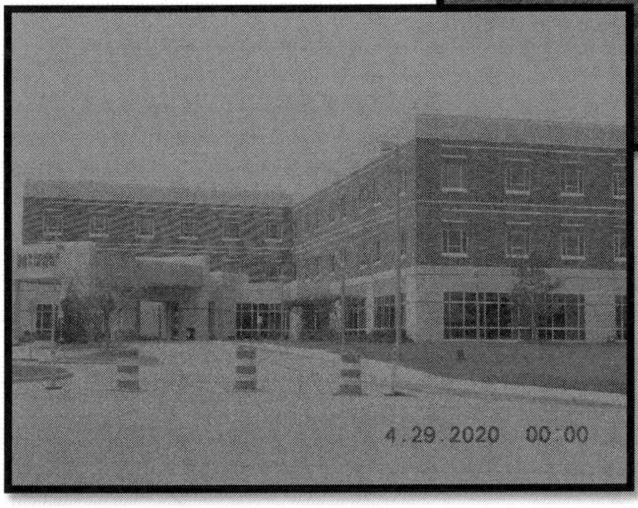

Figure 18 Banners lining the gates to Novant Hospital, Brunswick County, NC.

Figure 74 Novant Hospital, Brunswick County, NC.

89

In multiple hot spots such as New York City, despite cries of needing thousands of ventilators and other supplies, demands had not occurred and they have found themselves not needing the extra hospital beds set up, or the ships which were brought in with hundreds of beds and personnel. It is a good thing those higher than anticipated numbers had not occurred as of the end of April. Social distancing and the public responding so responsibly were touted as the reason.

The Thunderbirds and the Blue Angels Support First Responders and Hospital Workers in New York City

On the 28th of April 2020, the amazing Air Force Jets, the United States Air Force Thunderbirds and the United States Navy Blue Angels, flew over New York and into other states such as Pennsylvania, together, in formation, honoring the First Responders and hospital workers. Since everyone was supposed to be staying home, this was a frontline salute to say thank you to the medical workers for their work. Many rushed to their windows to watch those flights in awe and delight. While normally reserved for World Series games and the Fourth of July, this was a unique display to see both of the services planes flying together.

It was the sign and sight of America in action as a tribute to everyone, but especially to those who had given their lives and those who continued to serve. What a sight to see this symbol of strength and hope. This would continue for weeks in various parts of the nation.

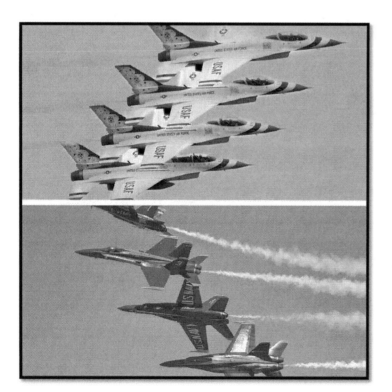

The effects of COVID-19 will go down in history as the global pandemic of 2020 that stopped the world. It literally, stopped the earth from shaking as it once did (due to travel and movement across the globe. The stay-at-home orders… stopped the world literally.

Figure 19 US Air Force Thunderbirds & US Navy Blue Angels.

90

The Sickness

People with a fever or cough were considered infectious and *testable* depending upon where they live, their travel history or other possible exposures. The entire U.S. was seeing some level of community spread of COVID-19. Testing for COVID-19 could be accessed through medical providers or public health departments, but there was no cure for this virus. Most people had mild illness and were able to recover at home without medical care. Others became deadly sick and needed a ventilator to breathe; especially those over 65 and those having severe underlying medical conditions. Those individuals were advised to take special precautions as they were at higher risk of developing serious complications and encouraged to basically quarantine at home.

Symptoms Associated with COVID-19

Risk depended upon characteristics of the virus, including how well it spread between people; the severity of resulting illness; and the medical or other measures available to control the impact of the virus (for example, vaccines or medications that can treat the illness) and the relative success of those. In the absence of vaccine or treatment medications, non-pharmaceutical interventions became the most important response strategy. These community interventions hoped to reduce the impact of disease.

There were (are) a variety of symptoms ranging from mild to severe. These appeared anywhere from 2 to 14 days after exposure to the virus. Among them are:

Fever or Chills	100.4 and up, Fahrenheit
Cough	Shortness of Breath/ Breathing Difficulties
Body Aches and Muscle Pains	Fatigue
Headache	New loss of taste or smell
Sore throat	Congestion or runny nose
Nausea or vomiting	Diarrhea

Children have similar symptoms to adults and generally had mild illness. Other less common symptoms were gastrointestinal symptoms like nausea, vomiting, or diarrhea. The following symptoms warranted an immediate trip to the hospital:

Trouble breathing	Persistent pain or pressure in the chest
New confusion	Inability to wake or stay awake
Bluish lips or face	

Collusion and Impeachment Proceedings

The COVID emergency was occurring at the same time as President Trump was being charged with collusion accusations, related to his election, and later impeachment charges by the House of Representatives in Washington, who were politically trying to have him removed from office through both processes. This eventually ended when the Senate voted against impeaching him and cleared him of all collusion charges. The content of those charges is beyond the scope of this text but readily available online. Here is how one American citizen felt at that time, in May of 2020.

Nina Blay of Pensacola, Florida

"As the USA was preparing for President Trump to be cleared (of all the collusion charges), once again, for the months leading up to his impeachment – we got sucker punched by the Pandemic COVID-19. It was a very scary time as we waited for further instructions about how to continue our lives. In our family, we were fortunate to have a long-planned wedding take place in Pensacola, Florida "just in time." "It was the week before our country started closing down and as I look back at the time of this beautiful wedding, I feel blessed and grateful that everyone, local and out-of-town guests, was there to celebrate with the couple," said Nina Blay of Pensacola, Florida.[46] She so succinctly summarized how the rest of us were feeling in mid-March 2020. That sucker punch still hurts in one way or another as our national communities continue to fight off the virus by August 2020.

May 9th –- Even the White House Staff is not Immune[47] 2020

The Coronavirus has now infected the White House. Reports declare that the Press Secretary for Vice President Mike Pence has tested positive for coronavirus. Katie Miller is 25 and tested positive this past Friday, yesterday.

In addition, the President's valet has tested positive. The White House Chief of Staff, Mark Meadows says, "They are taking more precautions."

Even Ivanka Trump's (President Trump's daughter) personal assistant has reportedly tested positive. Eleven Secret Service employees have also tested positive. Even the White House is not immune to this deadly and infectious disease.

---

[46] Blay, Nina. Pensacola, Florida. Comments on May 12, 2020.
[47] KTVU. Second White House staff member infected with coronavirus as President Trump shuns mask for VE Day ceremony. By Jana Katsuyam; Coronavirus KTVU FOX 2https://www.ktvu.com/news/second-white-house-staff-member-infected-with-coronavirus-as-president-trump-shuns-mask-for-ve-day-ceremony.

3 Top U.S. Officials Self-Quarantine After Potential COVID-19 Exposure[48]

After White House staff members tested positive for the coronavirus during the past few days, three more top U.S. health officials announced they are going into quarantine for the next two weeks, according to the Associated Press.

Anthony Fauci, MD, director of the National Institute of Allergy and Infectious Diseases, said on Saturday evening that he was beginning a "modified quarantine." Stephen Hahn, MD, commissioner of the FDA, and Robert Redfield, MD, director of the CDC, also said Saturday that they would begin a period of self-isolation.

All three are members of the White House coronavirus task force. They all tested negative on Friday, their corresponding institutions reported.

Fauci faces a "relatively low risk" due to minimal exposure to the staff member who tested positive, the news wire reported. He will work from home but go to the White House if needed.

Redfield also had "low risk exposure," the CDC said in a statement, and will telework for two weeks.

Hahn will also "self-quarantine" for two weeks, the FDA said.

The three health officials were slated to testify at a Senate committee hearing on Tuesday, according to Reuters. The committee is discussing ways that the states and federal government are reopening schools and businesses. The officials will receive a "one-time exception" to testify by videoconference, the committee said on Saturday evening. (One year later video conferencing and working from home became a new norm for many.)

The White House began testing Trump, Pence and other senior officials daily after Trump's valet tested positive.

Hahn came into contact with Miller, according to Politico. Miller coordinated communications among coronavirus task force members. The CDC and FDA didn't identify the person who tested positive and had contact with the health officials.

Other top health officials are monitoring the situation, the Washington Post reported. Alex Azar, secretary of Health and Human Services (HHS), tested negative on Friday and is "following the advice of his physicians at the White House Medical Unit," a spokeswoman told the newspaper. Brett Giroir, the assistant secretary for HHS, has participated in meetings remotely since Tuesday and has tested negative as well.

---

[48] WEB MD. https://www.webmd.com/lung/news/20200124/coronavirus-2020-outbreak-latest-updates. Web MD News Staff. May 10, 2020.

On Friday, White House staff members received a memo that encouraged employees to "practice maximum telework" and "work remotely if at all possible," the newspaper reported.

The memo said the White House will receive "heightened levels of daily cleaning" and that employees must report their travel.

"For any presumptive positive COVID-19 results, the White House medical unit conducts immediate contact tracing and notifies any affected individuals," the memo said. (Six months later, contact tracing became a standard practice across the nation, in an attempt to identify all potentially affected individuals and control the spread.)

May 10, 2020 Developments[49]

This virus continued to be more than anyone could mentally process.

Cases surpassed 117,000 worldwide; deaths exceeded 4,200.

Europe struggled to limit virus spread, led by the Italian lockdown.

Rational people are panic buying as coronavirus spreads.

Both leading candidates for the Democratic nomination canceled Tuesday events.

Turkey Has First Case, Puts Hospitals on Alert.

Sanders, Biden Scrap Planned Rallies.

FDA Suspends Inspections of Foreign Factories.

N.Y. to Close Gathering Places in NYC Suburb.

U.K. Outlines Easing Plans; South Korea Flare-Up: Virus Update.

Gilead's COVID-19 Drug Seen in Short Supply for Americans.

Japan Nears End to Its Loose Lockdown with Drop in Virus Cases.

Outbreak on North Korea Border Raises Doubts over its Virus Toll.

UN Closes New York Headquarters to Visitors.

St. Peter's Square, Basilica Closed to Tourists.

Spain Cases Topped 1,600.

---

[49] World Wide Web. May 10, 2020.

Cases of Remdesivir Shipped to Several States for COVID-19.

As Society Reopens, Not Everyone is Ready.

Evidence Mounts for Greater COVID Prevalence.

Blood Clots Are Another Dangerous COVID-19 Mystery.

The Great Invader: How COVID Attacks Every Organ.

Everyone continued to watch the statistics as they waited for their own individual states to decide how the latest federal guidelines would be implemented, how long each phase until re-opening will last, etc. They waited and waited and waited.

Flu Comparison[50]

Some people said COVID-19 was like the flu; was it?

The 10-year average of about **28,645,000** flu cases per year has a **1.6%** hospitalization rate and a **0.13%** mortality rate. Unfortunately, COVID-19 is currently **14 times** more deadly at **1.8%** with a **20%** overall hospitalization rate. There were 28,645,000 cases of COVID...however, but there are currently:

FLU HOSPITALIZATIONS- 458,320

TOTAL COVID-19 HOSPITALIZATIONS -5,729,000

TOTAL FLU DEATHS - 37,239   TOTAL COVID-19 DEATHS - 515,610

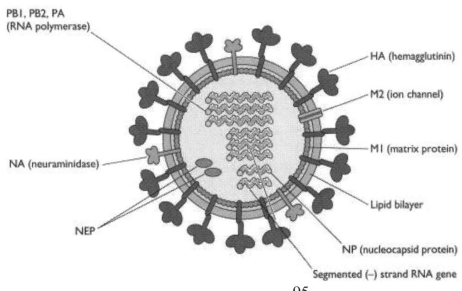

There was a big difference between the effects and spread of the flu and COVID.

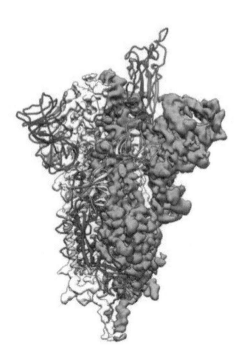

This is the 3D atomic scale map or molecular structure of the SARS-2-CoV protein "spike" which the virus uses to invade human cells. (Image credit: Jason McLellan/Univ. of Texas at Austin).[51]

Nope they are not alike.

———

Matthew 21:21-22 - And Jesus answered them, "Truly, I say to you, if you have faith and do not doubt, you will not only do what has been done to the fig tree, but even if you say to this mountain, 'Be taken up and thrown into the sea,' it will happen. And whatever you ask in prayer, you will receive, if you have faith."

---

[51] https://www.livescience.com/coronavirus-spike-protein-structure.html

Chapter 6

Covid-19 Globally

The world had been touched in nearly every country by this virus. Locations with confirmed COVID-19 cases, by WHO Region (World Health Organization) are documented with cases and deaths on May 10, 2020 in the following chart:[52]

229 Countries Reported

Total Global cases: 4,055,863   Total Deaths: 279,892

Country	Cases May 10, 2020	Deaths May 10, 2020
Abkhazia (aw)	3	1
Afghanistan	4,402	120
Albania	868	31
Algeria	5,723	502
Andorra	754	98
Angola	43	2
Angilla	3	0
Antigua & Barbuda	24	3
Argentina	5,763	300

---

[52] Global Case counts. Wikipedia. https://en.wikipedia.org/wiki/COVID-19_pandemic_by_country_and_territory#COVID19-container

Armenia	3,313	45
Artsakh	10	0
Aruba	101	3
Australia	6,927	97
Austria	15,786	618
Azerbaijan	2,422	31
Bahamas	92	11
Bahrain	4,856	8
Bangladesh	12,657	228
Barbados	84	7
Belarus	22,973	131
Belgium	53,081	8,656
Belize	18	2
Benin	319	2
Bermuda	118	7
Bhutan	7	0
Bolivia	2,437	114
Bonaired	2	0
Bosnia & Herzegovina	2,117	107
Botswana	23	1
Brazil	156,604	10,697
British Virgin Islands	7	1
Brunei	141	1
Bulgaria	1965	91
Burkina Faso	748	48
Burundi	15	1
Cambodia	122	0

Cameroon	2,579	114
Canada	68,003	4,728
Cape Verde	236	2
Cayman Islands	81	1
Central African Republic	143	0
Chad	322	31
Charles de Gaulle	1,081	0
Chile	28,866	13,112
China	82,901	4,633
Columbia	10,495	445
Comoros	11	1
Congo	274	10
Coral	12	2
Costa Atlantica	148	0
Costa Rica	780	6
Croatia	2,187	90
Cuba	1,754	74
Curacao	16	1
Cyprus	892	15
Czech Republic	8,095	276
DR Congo	937	39
Denmark	10,429	529
Diamond Princess	712	14
Djibouti	1,189	3
Dolfijn	8	0
Cominica	16	0
Dominican Republic	10,347	388

Donetsk PR	180	5
East Timor	24	0
Ecuador	289,071	1,717
Egypt	3,964	514
El Salvador	889	17
Equatorial Guinea	439	4
Eritrea	39	0
Estonia	1,739	60
Eswatini	163	2
Ethiopia	239	5
Falkland Islands	13	0
Faroe Islands	187	0
Fiji	18	0
Finland	5,962	267
France	138,854	26,310
French Polynesia	60	0
Gabon	661	8
Georgia	635	10
Germany	171,539	7,549
Ghana	4,263	7,549
Ghana	4,263	22
Gibraltar	146	0
Greece	2,710	151
Greenland	11	0
Greg Mortimer	128	0
Grenada	21	0
Guam	151	5

Guatemala	967	24
Guernsey	252	13
Guinea	2,042	11
Guinea-Bissau	641	3
Guyana	97	10
Haiti	151	12
Honduras	1,830	108
Hong Kong	1,048	4
Hungary	3,263	413
Iceland	1,801	10
India	62,939	2,109
Indonesia	14,032	973
Iran	107,603	6,640
Iraq	2,679	107
Ireland	22,760	1,446
Isle of Man	330	23
Israel	16,458	248
Italy	218,268	30,395
Ivory Coast	1,667	21
Jamaica	498	9
Japan	15,777624	
Jersey	293	25
Jordan	522	9
Kazakhstan	5,076	31
Kenya	672	32
Kosovo	870	28
Kuwait	8,688	58

Kyrgyzstan	1,002	12
Laos	19	0
Latvia	939	18
Lebanon	845	26
Liberia	199	20
Libya	64	3
Liechtenstein	82	1
Lithuania	1,479	50
Luhansk PR	232	2
Luxembourg	3,877	101
Macau	45	0
Madagascar	193	0
Malawi	56	3
Malaysia	6,656	108
Maldives	835	3
Mali	692	37
Malta	496	5
Mauritania	8	1
Mauritius	332	10
Mexico	33,460	3,353
Moldova	4,867	161
Monaco	96	4
Mongolia	42	0
Montenegro	324	9
Montserrat	11	1
Morocco	6,038	188
Mozambique	91	0

Myanmar	180	6
Namibia	16	0
Nepal	110	0
Netherlands	42,627	5,440
New Caledonia	18	0
New Zealand	1,144	21
Nicaragua	16	5
Niger	815	45
Nigeria	4,151	128
Macedonia	1,642	128
Cyprus	108	4
Mariana Islands	15	2
Norway	8,099	219
Oman	3,399	17
Pakistan	29,465	8,023
Palestine	375	4
Panama	8,282	237
Guinea	8	0
Paraguay	689	10
Peru	65,015	1,814
Philippines	10,794	719
Poland	15,821	618
Portugal	27,581	1,135
Puerto Rico	2,198	111
Qatar	22,520	14
Romania	15,362	952
Russia	209,688	1,915

Rwanda	280	O
Saba	2	0
Saint Kitts & Nevis	15	0
Saint Lucia	18	0
Saint Pierre & Miquelon	1	0
Saint Vincent	17	0
San Marino	637	41
Sao Tome & Principe	208	5
Saudi Arabia	39,048	246
Senegal	1,709	18
Serbia	10,114	213
Seychelles	11	0
Sierra Leone	307	18
Singapore	23,336	20
Sint Eustatius	2	0
Sint Maarten	76	15
Slovakia	1,457	26
Slovenia	1,457	102
Somalia	1,054	51
Somali Land	6	0
South Africa	9,420	186
South Korea	10,874	256
South Ossetia	3	0
South Sudan	120	0
Spain	224,390	26,621
Sri Lanka	856	9
Sudan	1,164	64

Suriname	10	1
Sweden	26,322	3,225
Switzerland	30,305	1,538
Syria	47	3
Taiwan	440	6
Tajikistan	612	20
Tanzania	509	21
Thailand	3,009	56
The Gambia	20	1
USS Theodore Roosevelt	1,102	1
Trinidad & Tobago	116	8
Tunisia	1,032	45
Turkey	138,657	3,786
Turks & Caicos Islands	12	1
U.S. Virgin Islands	69	4
Uganda	116	0
Ukraine	15,232	391
United Arab Emirates	18,198	198
United Kingdom	219,183	31,855
United States	1,351,225	80,001
Uruguay	702	18
Uzbekistan	2,411	10
Vatican City	12	0
Venezuela	402	10
Vietnam	288	0
Yemen	34	7
Zaandam	4	13

Zambia	252	7
Zimbabwe	36	4

As of 10 May 2020 (UTC) ·

History of cases: China, international.

•This number shows the cumulative number of confirmed human cases reported to date. The actual number of infections and cases is likely to be higher than reported.

•The total number of cases may not necessarily add up due to the frequency of values being updated for each location.

•Reporting criteria and testing capacity varies between countries.

•Countries, territories, and international conveyances where cases were diagnosed. The nationality of the infected and the origin of infection may vary. For some countries, cases are split into respective territories and noted accordingly.

•Total deaths may not necessarily add up due to the frequency of values updating for each location. Reporting criteria varies between countries.

United States - Figures include cases identified on the Grand Princess. -Figures do not include the unincorporated territories of Puerto Rico, Guam, Northern Mariana Islands, and U.S. Virgin Islands, all of which are listed separately. -Cases include clinically diagnosed cases as per CDC guidelines. -Recoveries and deaths include probable deaths and people released from quarantine as per CDC guidelines. -Figures from the United States Department of Defense are only released on a branch-by branch basis since April 2020, without distinction between domestic and foreign deployment, and cases may be reported to local health authorities. -Cases for the USS Theodore Roosevelt, currently docked at Guam, are reported separate from national figures but included in the Navy's totals. -There is also one case reported from Guantanamo Bay Naval Base not included in any other nation or territory's counts. Since April 2020, the United States Department of Defense has directed all bases, including Guantanamo Bay, to not publicize case statistics.

Spain - Excludes serology–confirmed cases.

United Kingdom - Excluding all British Overseas Territories and Crown dependencies.

Russia - -Including cases from the disputed Crimea and Sevastopol. -Excluding the cases from Diamond Princess cruise ship which are classified as "on an international conveyance".

France - Including French overseas regions Saint Martin and Saint Barthélemy. -Excluding collectivities of New Caledonia, French Polynesia and Saint Pierre and Miquelon. -Figures for total confirmed cases and total deaths include data from both hospital and nursing homes.

China - Excluding 794 asymptomatic cases under medical observation as of 9 May 2020. - Asymptomatic cases were not reported before 31 March 2020. -Excluding Special Administrative Regions of Hong Kong and Macau. Does not include Taiwan.

Belgium - The number of deaths also includes untested cases and cases in retirement homes that presumably died   because of COVID-19, whilst most countries only include deaths of tested cases in hospitals.

Netherlands - All four constituent countries of the Kingdom of the Netherlands (i.e. the country of the Netherlands [in this table row], Aruba, Curaçao, and Sint Maarten) and the special municipalities of the Caribbean Netherlands (Bonaire, Saba and Sint Eustatius) are listed separately.

Chile - -Including the special territory of Easter Island. -On 29 April 2020, the Chilean government started to inform the number of asymptomatic confirmed cases, separated from the official number of confirmed cases. Since 30 April, all confirmed cases (no matter their symptoms) are included in the official number. -Chilean authorities define a person as "recovered" after 14 days since the detection of the virus because "they are no longer contagious". Initially, patients who have died of coronavirus were counted as recovered, following the same criteria, according to Health Minister Jaime Mañalich; however, this was changed later and Chilean reports inform the number of recovered separated from the deceased.

Israel - -Including cases from the disputed Golan Heights. -Excluding cases from the State of Palestine. -Diamond Princess and Japan. -The British cruise ship Diamond Princess was in Japanese waters, and the Japanese administration was asked to manage its quarantine, with the passengers having not entered Japan. Therefore, this case is included in neither the Japanese nor British official counts. The World Health Organization classifies the cases as being located "on an international conveyance."

Ukraine - -Excluding cases from the disputed Crimea and Sevastopol. Cases in these territories are included in the Russian total. -Excluding cases from the unrecognized Donetsk and Lugansk People's Republics.

Denmark - -The autonomous territories of the Faroe Islands and Greenland are listed separately.

Serbia - Excluding cases from the disputed Kosovo.

Egypt - Includes cases identified on the MS River Anuket.

Norway - Estimation of the number of infected: -As of 23 March 2020, according to figures from just over 40 per cent of all GPs in Norway, 20,200 patients have been registered with the "corona code" R991. The figure includes both cases where the patient has been diagnosed with coronavirus infection through testing, and where the GP has used the "corona code" after assessing the patient's symptoms against the criteria by the Norwegian Institute of Public Health. -As of 24 March 2020, the Norwegian Institute of Public Health estimates that between 7,120 and 23,140 Norwegians are infected with the coronavirus.

Australia -Excluding the cases from Diamond Princess cruise ship which are classified as "on an international conveyance". Ten cases, including one fatality recorded by the Australian government.

Morocco -Including cases in the disputed Western Sahara territory controlled by Morocco. There are no confirmed cases in the rest of Western Sahara.

Finland -Including the autonomous region of the Åland Islands.

Argentina -Excluding confirmed cases on the claimed territory of the Falkland Islands. Since 11 April, the Argentine Ministry of Health includes them in their official reports.

Moldova -Including the disputed territory of Transnistria.

Azerbaijan -Excluding the self-declared state of Artsakh.

Cuba -Includes cases on the MS Braemar. -Excluding cases from Guantanamo Bay, which is governed by the United States.

New Zealand -Guam and USS Theodore Roosevelt

-Cases for the USS Theodore Roosevelt, currently docked at Guam, are reported separately.

Charles de Gaulle -Including cases on the escort frigate Chevalier Paul. -Florence Parly, Minister of the Armed Forces, reported to the National Assembly's National Defense and Armed Forces Committee that 2010 sailors of the carrier battle group led by Charles de Gaulle had been tested, with 1081 tests returning positive so far. Many of these cases were aboard Charles de Gaulle, some of the cases were reportedly aboard French frigate Chevalier Paul, and it is unclear if any other ships in the battle group had cases on board.

Somalia -Excluding the de facto state of Somaliland.

DR Congo -The Democratic Republic of the Congo.

Cyprus -Including the British Overseas Territory of Akrotiri and Dhekelia. -Excluding de facto state of Northern Cyprus.

Greg Mortimer and Uruguay -Although currently anchored off the coast of Uruguay, cases for the Greg Mortimer are currently reported separately. Six have been transferred inland for hospitalization.

Georgia -Excluding the de facto state of Abkhazia.

Taiwan -Including cases from the ROCS Pan Shi.

Congo -Also known as the Republic of the Congo and not to be confused with the DR Congo.

Donetsk and Luhansk People's Republic -Note that these territories are distinct from the Ukraine-administered regions of the Donetsk and Luhansk Oblasts.

Northern Cyprus -Cases from this de facto state are not counted by Cyprus.

Syria -Excluding cases from the disputed Golan Heights.   Saint Vincent. -The sovereign state of Saint Vincent and the Grenadines.

MS Zaandam -Including cases from MS Rotterdam. -The MS Rotterdam rendezvoused with the Zaandam on March 26 off the coast of Panama City to provide support and evacuate healthy passengers. Both have since docked in Florida.   -MS Zaandam and Rotterdam's numbers are currently not counted in any national figures.

Artsakh -Cases from this de facto state are not counted by Azerbaijan.

HNLMS Dolfijn -All 8 cases currently associated with Dolfijn were reported while the submarine was at sea in the waters between Scotland and the Netherlands. -It is unclear whether the Netherlands National Institute for Public Health and the Environment (RIVM) is including these cases in their total count, but neither their daily update details nor their daily epidemiological situation reports appear to have mentioned the ship, with a breakdown of cases listing the twelve provinces of the country of the Netherlands (as opposed to the kingdom) accounting for all the cases in the total count.

Somaliland -Cases from this de facto state are not counted by Somalia.

Abkhazia -Cases from this de facto state are not counted by Georgia.

South Ossetia -Cases from this de facto state are not counted by Georgia.

The Story in Uganda

The Corona Virus was late getting started in most of Africa according to media information. By the end of April 2020, it had pretty much spread to all of the countries listed in the preceding chart.

Tusiime Katogi Ronald, a police dog trainer and security company owner, described his experiences with the virus in Kampala City, Uganda, with the following:

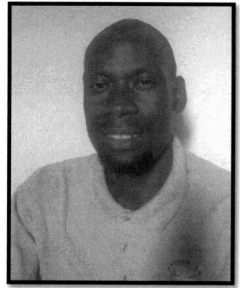
Figure 20 Tusiime Ronald.

"The breaking news from here is that a certain man has eaten a Chameleon as a potential vaccine against the COVID-19. He is now under medical supervision," he said chuckling.

Getting serious, he went on to explain that "the food markets are open with the vendors camping there at the markets overnight. They are not allowed to travel back and forth to their homes to avoid spreading the virus from there to their family. Pictures from the newspaper, the *Daily Monitor,* showed vendors camping in what appears to be mosquito net type tents."

"There is no transport for anyone, no busses or other means. Patients are being taken to the hospital on homemade wooden wheel barrows as printed in the Kampala City newspaper, *The Monitor."* "A lady with a broken leg had a homemade wheel barrow as her taxi in the municipality of Arua. She could not access a boda boda a common means of transportation there, following a ban on public transport," he said.

Ronald went on to describe their situation with, "The government is distributing food; mostly beans and maize flour, to the most vulnerable groups. These folks survive on their daily bread. However, my family is not provided with those supplies. There does not seem to be enough to go around."

The UGANDA Presidential Guidelines to Manage the Spread of the Coronavirus, posted April 2020, listed the following:

Suspended

⊛Movements in and out of country for 32 days.

⊛Public Transport for 14 days.

⊛Private transport for 14 days.

⊛Boda Bodas for 14 days. Boda bodas are bicycles and motorcycles used as taxis in East Africa.

⊛Tuk-Tuks for 14 days. (a three-wheeled motorized vehicle in Southeast Asia and some parts of Africa and South America.

⊛Coaches for 14 days.

⊛Buses for 14 days.

⊛Air Transport for 32 days.

Mr. Yoweri Museveni had been the President of Uganda since 29 January 1986. He went on to prohibit:

⊛Gatherings of more than 5 people.   ⊛Parties.

⊛Bars.   ⊛Communal weddings.

⊛Political rallies and events.   ⊛Movements of any form between 7:00 pm and 6:30 am.

Food

⊛Government will provide food for those affected.

Government Workers

⊛Stay home.

⊛Army, the Police, the Health workers, the Electricity, Water and Telephone workers allowed.

⊛People in barracks should not get out.

Closed

⊛Shopping malls for 14 days.   ⊛Arcades for 14 days.

⊛Hardware shops for 14 days.   ⊛Lodges for 14 days.

⊛Salons for 14 days.   ⊛Non-Food stores for 14 days.

⊛Non-food markets for 32 days.   ⊛Garages for 14 days.

Allowed (with Precautions)

⊛Food Markets – 4 metres circumferential distance, workers must stay at the camp.

⊛Supermarkets-Regulate numbers that come and leave.

⊛Construction sites: workers must stay at camp.

⊛Factories-workers must camp.

⊛Pharmacies   ⊛Vet Shops   ⊛Agric stores

⊛Banks   ⊛Judiciary   ⊛Media houses

⊛Private companies   ⊛Garbage collection services

⊛Fuel Stations   ⊛Water departments

⊛KCCA staff   ⊛Telecommunication

⊛Door-to-door delivery   ⊛Cleaning services

⊛Medical centres   ⊛Agriculture

Business

⊛URA shall not close businesses on account of not paying taxes during these 14 days.

⊛Cargo transport must continue.

⊛No disconnection of WATER and ELECTRICITY during this time.

⊛No seizing properties due to non-loan payment.

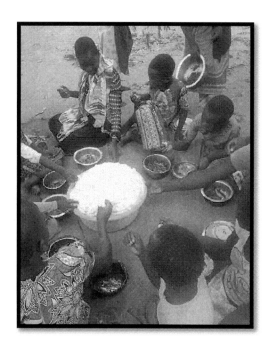

Security and Health

⊛The vehicles of the Army, Police, ambulances, utilities, vehicles, Prisons, UWA, etc., will continue to move on orders of the competent authorities.

⊛Government cars to help deliver people to hospital.

Curfew 7:00 pm to 6:30 am.

Figure 21 Daily meals in Uganda during the lockdown. Photograph courtesy of Tusiime Ronald.

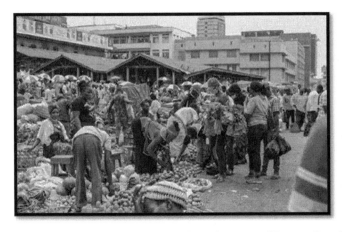

Figure 22Uganda Food Markets. Photo Courtesy of Tusiime Ronald.

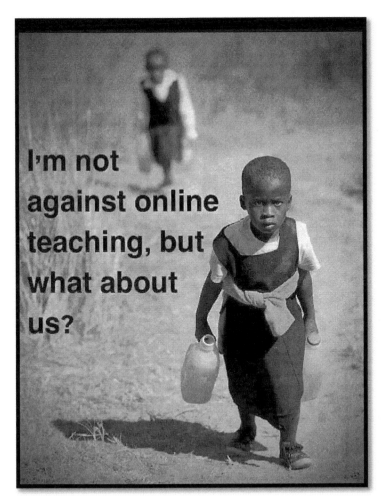

I'm not against online teaching, but what about us?

When asked about his personal family (Tusiime Ronald), he said, "My family is fine. No virus. Everyone in the country is under quarantine so they stay home. For food, we send motorcycle taxis to pick up and deliver to us." He went on to say, "We are told that some patients have recovered and are back in their homes." However, when questioned further, he stated, "Well, we are struggling. Some time ago I bought corn and bean seeds. We are eating that at this time." "It seems that the governments' promise to distribute maize flour and green beans only goes as far as the most vulnerable, and medical and state workers. None seems to be available for the families in the small villages."

Figure 23 Uganda children.

Figure 24 Kabale Regional Referral Hospital.

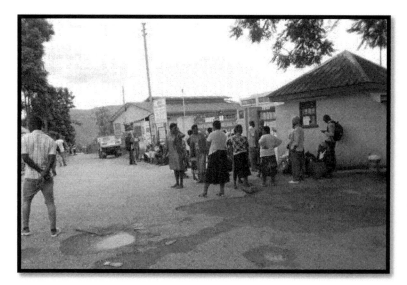

"Mothers are stranded at the Kabale Regional Referral Hospital. They were discharged but they cannot go home because of transport. Nobody is there to rescue them. Imagine a woman who has given birth through Caesarian section trekking 15 kilometers to get home…"[53]

When Tusiime K. Ronald was asked if he sees a Chinese presence in Africa, he stated that, "We only see many Chinese investors here controlling most industries and factories. They are building roads, businesses and many other things." When asked if he had heard anything about many millions of Chinese destined to be sent to Africa, he responded, "No, as our leaders hide much from us." Earlier this year, Chinese officers took command of a Zambian police force for unpaid debt. Is this the method used by China to take over Africa? That would be a topic for another book. Time will show what happens in Uganda and other African countries with the influx of the Chinese yen.

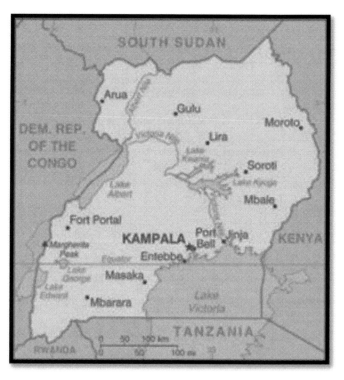

---

[53] Charles Rwomushana says Under M7…#Mpawo Atalikaba.Uganda.

114

On April 21, 2020, there were the following confirmed cases as reported by the local newspaper in Uganda, the *Daily Monitor*[54]:

Confirmed Cases in Africa

Tanzania-284   Kenya-303

Uganda-61   Rwanda-147

Italy

Video Captures Gliding Jellyfish Visible in Venice's Canals as Italy Remains on Lockdown

"As tourists stay home during the ongoing coronavirus pandemic, Venice has become quiet. The boat traffic that normally fills the canals has dramatically lessened the waterways; criss-crossing the city have noticeably cleared. Mangoni told Reuters that the low tide and low traffic due to Italy's ongoing travel restrictions made it possible to observe marine life right in the center of the normally boisterous city."[55] April 22, 2020.

Russia

Moscow's coronavirus offensive[56]

ROME — As the coronavirus spreads, Russia appears to be observing the adage that you should never let a good crisis go to waste.

Seeking to capitalize on the chaos and promote its own soft power, the Kremlin has taken Beijing's lead and started love-bombing struggling nations with medical aid, and stepping up its efforts to broadcast propaganda and sow disinformation on state and social media.

In March, medical supplies airlifted to Italy were emblazoned with the logo "From Russia with Love." Even more surreal was Russia's deployment of 122 experts in bacterial warfare, including medical teams, to Italy.

---

[54] Source: Ministries of Health • Last Updated: 21/04/2020
[55] Time. Melissa Locker. Time. April 22, 2020. https://news.yahoo.com/video-captures-gliding-jellyfish-visible-150742865.html.
[56] Politico. By Hannah Roberts. Politico. April 21, 2020. https://news.yahoo.com/moscow-coronavirus-offensive-025611769.html.

Scenes of the convoy of 22 military trucks, rolling across Italy like an occupying power, constituted a propaganda coup for Moscow, which used the images to hammer home the idea that NATO and the European Union have abandoned Italy in its hour of need. "Russian convoy traveled on NATO roads," state-controlled Rossiya 1 TV channel crowed.

A video of an Italian man taking down an EU flag and replacing it with a Russian tricolor and a sign saying "Thank you Putin" has played frequently on Russian TV — no matter that Italian media later reported people had of received payments of €200 for filming messages of gratitude.

Outside Italy, Russia has also dispatched help to hard-hit countries within its sphere of influence, such as Serbia and Belarus, and sold much-needed medical supplies to the U.S., welcomed by President Donald Trump.

The tactic is familiar, and fits into a broader effort to undermine trust in the Western liberal order. But the PR moves also serve another, perhaps more important, purpose: At home, the tactic diverts attention from an explosion of cases within Russia's own borders and boosts domestic perceptions of President Vladimir Putin's statesmanship on the international stage.

By sending aid to another country, Russia is seeking to redraw global hierarchies, said Raffaele Marchetti, a professor of international relations at Luiss University in Rome. April 21, 2020.

Sweden

Unlike most of the world, Sweden decided *not* to impose restrictions on its citizens. Restaurants have remained open, cafes are full, and playgrounds are still open. The rest of the world watches as their ideas about promoting the group immunity concept once everyone catches it, known as the *herd immunity*. As of mid-April the infection rate was rising with about 150 deaths per one million people. This is a death rate which is higher than neighboring countries. They are building field hospitals as well. Sweden is confident that the death rate is peaking and their herd immunity plan will work in the long run. It did not happen.

Philippines

Jeffrey Lee Rafael Juntoria, a resident of Barangay Tuburan Pototan, Iloilo City, Philippines, described the situation in the Philippines in his town like this: "When Corona virus hit the Philippines, it was the start of total chaos."

"City per city went on lockdown. No one is allowed to go out of their houses. No one is allowed to go astray. Curfews have been implemented and social distancing has been strictly followed. Everyone is asked to sanitize and stay home."

The Manilla Reuters reported that as of May 3, 2020 the number of cases of corona rose to 9,223 with a rise of 295 infections on Sunday; yesterday. The minister of health reports the death toll at 607 as of this date.

He continued by saying, "Day by day, the virus spread and has become rampant. Fast as the light. There is not a day that passes with no casualties. The death toll is raised hour by hour. The number of people infected grows by numbers. This has caused the *Enhanced Community Quarantine* to be implemented. At this time, no one can go outside of their house."

Because of the shortage of masks, some Filipinos, like others around the world, created their own like Juvy Juntoria.

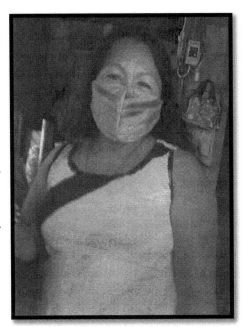

Figure 25 Map of the Philippines.

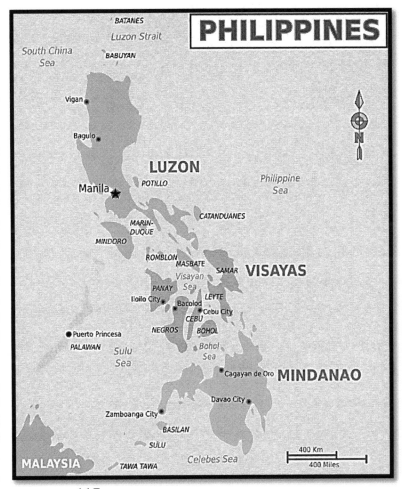

Every household was granted one Quarantine Pass. One member of the household could do all the chores that needed to be done outside the home such as going to the market, buying things, etc.," Jeffrey Juntoria said. "In order to go to the market, one has to be scheduled. Village by village should go to the market on its designated day of the week. You cannot just simply go there and do your grocery shopping anytime or day you want."

Juntoria stated that, "Liquor has been banned as well. But people are sneaking alcoholic drinks just to be able to have a taste of it at night. Boredom strikes everyone.

117

Above all, the fear of the virus lives within the hearts of every Filipino."

"The Quarantine started March 14, 2020 and originally it was supposed to end by April 14th but has been extended until the 30th of April. Now they plan to extend it until the 15th of May." (Noted on April 24, 2020) Juntoria said, "It is hard for people who make a living by going out of their houses every day. There is some food assistance but it will not suffice. Everybody stopped working except for the front-liners: the police, army, the public servants, and those working in the hospitals. A lot of front-liners have taken their last breath rendering service to the people. Many have died of the COVID-19. This pandemic situation is sucking the life of Filipinos day-by-day. This is not just another virus with an antidote. This one has none yet and no cure." Juntoria said, "People are extending help in any way possible. It may be by providing food or monetary, or crops; anything that could be of help to fellow citizens. Yes, we have experienced and are experiencing hardships brought on by this pandemic, COVID-19. This has made us stronger, wiser and we have learned to appreciate everything that we have. I must say, lessons are really learned the hard way. Yet we will not be stopped by just a virus. We are still hoping, that the day will come when we will open our eyes from a deep sleep to find a bright sunny morning; and everything will be back to normal. We are yearning for this dark chapter of our lives to be closed and a new one to unfold with hearts full of hope and smiles on our faces. And we will utter, "Thank you God, for the gift of life. Thank you for giving us another shot at life; and continue to live."

World Health Organization Situational Global Report - May 9, 2020[57]

Australia reported a total of 6,927 cases and 97 deaths.

Belarus recorded a total of 21,101 cases and 26 deaths.

Canada reported 157 new deaths, bringing the death toll to 4,628. Canada has reported 1,381 cases, bringing the total to 66,780.

France reported 80 deaths, bringing the death toll to 26,310. 22,614 remain in hospital with 2,812 in intensive care.

Germany reported 1,251 cases, bringing the total to 168,551. Germany has reported 147 deaths, bringing the death toll to 7,369.

Indonesia reported 533 new cases, bringing the total to 13,645. Indonesia has reported 16 deaths, bringing the total to 959.

---

[57] Timelines of the COVID-19 Pandemic in May of 2020. Wikipedia.
https://en.wikipedia.org/wiki/Timeline_of_the_COVID-19_pandemic_in_May_2020. May 9 – 11.

Iran reported 1,529 new cases, bringing the total to 106,220. Iran has reported 48 deaths, bringing the death toll to 6,589. While most provinces have seen a drop in cases, cases have continued to rise in Khuzestan.

Italy reported 194 deaths, bringing the death toll to 30,395. Italy has reported 1,083 new cases, bringing the total to 218,268. 1,034 remain in intensive care.

Malaysia reported 54 new cases, bringing the total to 6,589. Malaysia has reported one death, bringing the total to 108.

New Zealand reported two new cases (one confirmed and the other probable), bringing the total to 1,492 (1,142 confirmed and 350 probable). 21 new recoveries have been reported, bringing the total to 1,368.

The Philippines reported 147 cases, bringing the total to 10,610. The Philippines has reported 8 deaths, bringing the total to 704.

Qatar reported 1,130 cases, bringing the total to 21,331. Qatar has reported one death, bringing the death toll to 13.

Russia reported 10,817 cases, bringing the total to 198,676. Russia has reported 104 deaths, bringing the death toll to 1,827.

Singapore reported 753 new cases, bringing the total to 22,460.

South Korea reported 18 new cases, bringing the total to 10,840. The country has reported 256 deaths.

Spain reported 721 new cases, bringing the total to 223,578. Spain has also reported 179 deaths, bringing the total to 26,478.

Thailand reported four new cases, bringing the total to 3,004. Thailand has also reported one death, bringing the death toll to 56.

Ukraine reported 515 new cases and 15 new deaths, bringing the total numbers to 14,710 and 376 respectively; a total of 2,909 patients have recovered.

The United Kingdom reported 346 deaths, bringing the death toll to 31,587.

The United States reported a total of 1,342,329 cases, 79,906 deaths, and 232,821 recoveries.[66] In New York, Governor Andrew Cuomo has announced that three more children have died of an infectious disease linked to COVID-19.

May 10

Brazil reported a total of 10,627 deaths and 155,939 cases. However, scientists believe that the real figures are higher due to a lack of widespread testing.

Canada reported 100 new deaths, bringing the death toll to 4,728. Canada has reported 1,216 new cases, bringing the total to 66,796.

China reported 14 new cases (12 community transmissions and 2 imported); 11 of these cases occurred in Jilin province and one in Hubei.

France reported 70 new deaths, bringing the death toll to 26,380. 36 people have been discharged from intensive care, bringing the total number in intensive care down to 2,776.

Germany reported 667 new cases, bringing the total to 169,218. Germany has also reported 26 deaths, bringing the death toll to 7,395.

Iran reported 51 new deaths.

Lebanon reported 36 new cases, bringing the total to 845. Lebanon's death toll remains at 26.

Malaysia reported 67 new cases (49 of them foreigners), bringing the total to 6,656. 1,525 remain in hospital; 18 in intensive care and 6 on ventilators. 96 have been discharged, bringing the total number of recoveries to 5,025. The death toll remains at 108.

New Zealand reported two new cases (both confirmed), bringing the total to 1,494 (1,144 confirmed and 350 probable). Two people remain in hospital. Three people have recovered, bringing the total to 1,371.

The Philippines reported 184 new cases, bringing the total to 10,794. 15 deaths have been recorded, bringing the death toll to 719. 82 have recovered, bringing the total number of recovered to 1,924.

Russia reported 11,012 new cases, bringing the total to 209,668. Russia has reported 88 deaths, bringing the death toll to 1,195.

Singapore reported 876 new cases, bringing the total to 23,336. In addition, 33 false positive tests were recorded due to calibration issues in one of the test kits.

South Korea reported 34 new cases (26 community transmissions and eight imported). Most of these cases have been linked to night clubs in Seoul's Itaewon district.

Spain reported 143 deaths, bringing the death toll to 26,621. Spain has reported 224,390 casualties.

Thailand reported five new cases, bringing the total to 3,009. The death toll remains at 59.

Turkey reported a total of 137,115 cases and 3,739 deaths.

Ukraine reported 522 new cases and 15 new deaths, bringing the total numbers to 15,232 and 391 respectively; a total of 2,909 patients have recovered.

The **United Kingdom** reported 269 deaths, bringing the national death toll to 31,855.

In the **United States**, at least 25,600 residents and workers have died at nursing homes and other long-term care facilities for the elderly. The coronavirus has affected 143,000 people at about 7,500 facilities.

A total of about 4 million cases, almost 1.4 million recoveries, and over 279,000 deaths have been reported globally.

May 11, 2020

Malaysia reported 70 new cases, bringing the total to 6,726. There are 1,504 active cases, with 20 cases in intensive care. 88 have been discharged, bringing the total number of recovered to 5,113. Malaysia has reported one new death, bringing the death toll to 109.

New Zealand reported three new cases (all confirmed), bringing the total to 1,497 (1,147 confirmed and 350 probable). 15 new recoveries have been reported, bringing the total to 1,386. The number of active cases has dropped below 90.

Singapore reported 486 new cases, bringing the total to 23,822.

Ukraine reported 416 new cases and 17 new deaths, bringing the total numbers to 15,648 and 408 respectively; a total of 3,288 patients have recovered.

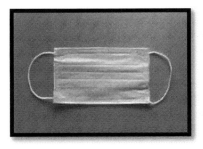

Global Cases March 19, 2021

Cases - cumulative total: **121,464,666**   Cases - newly reported in last 24 hours - **535,860**

Deaths - cumulative total - **2,684,093**   Deaths - newly reported in last 24 hours - **9,868**

Country	Cases	New Cases	Deaths	Deaths last 24 hrs
United States	29,317,562	56,790	532,971	1,116
Brazil	11,693,838	90,303	284,775	2,648
India	11,514,331	39,726	159,370	154
Russian Federation	4,437,938	9,699	94,267	443
The United Kingdom	4,280,886	6,303	125,926	95
France	4,111,105	34,936	91,162	269
Italy	3,306,711	24,901	103,855	423
Spain	3,206,116	0	72,793	0
Turkey	2,950,603	20,049	29,777	81
Germany	2,629,750	17,482	74,358	22
Colombia	2,314,154	4,554	61,498	130
Argentina	2,218,425	8,304	54,231	195
Mexico	2,175,462	6,455	195,908	789
South Africa	1,533,961	1,464	51,724	90
Ukraine	1,519,926	15,850	29,515	262
Czechia	1,449,696	10,677	24,331	214
Indonesia	1,443,853	6,570	39,142	227
Peru	1,435,598	7,994	49,523	193
Netherlands	1,179,612	6,187	16,198	33
Canada	919,239	3,371	22,554	35
Chile	911,469	6,257	21,988	172
Romania	881,159	6,174	21,877	90
Israel	824,716	1,517	6,064	12
Belgium	822,801	1	22,624	4
Portugal	816,055	485	16,743	21
Iraq	779,458	5,443	13,896	36
Sweden	738,537	6,442	13,236	1

Philippines	640,984	5,286	12,887	21
Pakistan	615,810	3,495	13,717	61
Switzerland	576,160	3	9,438	0
Bangladesh	564,939	2,187	8,624	16
Hungary	549,839	10,759	17,841	213
Serbia	536,904	5,346	4,840	30
Jordan	514,107	9,192	5,627	74
Austria	501,387	3,505	8,770	23
Morocco	490,575	487	8,748	3
Japan	452,702	1,516	8,758	41
United Arab Emirates	434,465	2,101	1,424	10
Lebanon	430,734	3,757	5,609	73
Saudi Arabia	383,880	381	6,591	6
Panama	349,020	440	6,018	9
Slovakia	346,149	1,679	8,894	80
Malaysia	328,466	1,213	1,223	3
Ecuador	307,429	1,831	16,333	33
Belarus	306,524	1,254	2,130	9
Bulgaria	295,777	4,008	11,817	102
Kazakhstan	277,906	0	3,511	0
Georgia	276,796	360	3,683	9
Nepal	275,625	107	3,015	1
Saba	6	0	0	0
Samoa	4	0	0	0
Marshall Islands	4	0	0	0
Vanuatu	3	0	0	0

NO CASES

Turkmenistan Tonga   Tokelau   Pitcairn Islands

Palau   Niue   Nauru

Micronesia (Federated States of)   Kiribati

Democratic People's Republic of Korea

Cook Islands

American Samoa

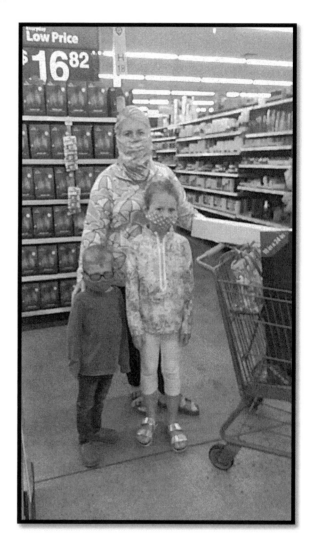

Figure 26 Shoppers at Walmart, Shallotte, NC.[58]

---

[58] Mrs. Whitney Traverson and her children Lacey and Luke shop at Walmart, Shallotte, NC. Residents of Bolivia, NC. April 23, 2020.

Chapter 7

Life with the Covid-19 Pandemic

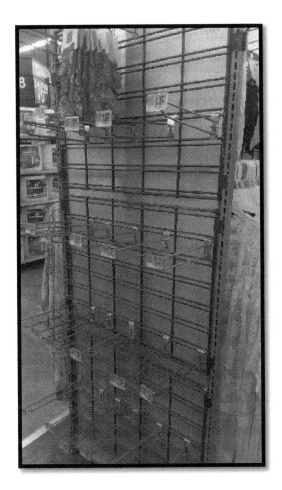

Figure 27 Shelf Empty of Bandanas.

On a typical day (April 23, 2020) of running errands, the Traverson family was observed with the entire family masked. At that particular trip, critical shelves were bare at Walmart in Shallotte, North Carolina. The bandana shelf was empty along with the paper goods aisles. No toilet paper could be found; a common occurrence since this virus began which precipitated unreasonable hoarding of certain supplies. In addition, antibacterial soap and cleaning products remained a valued commodity, more often than not, absent from the store shelves.

Masks

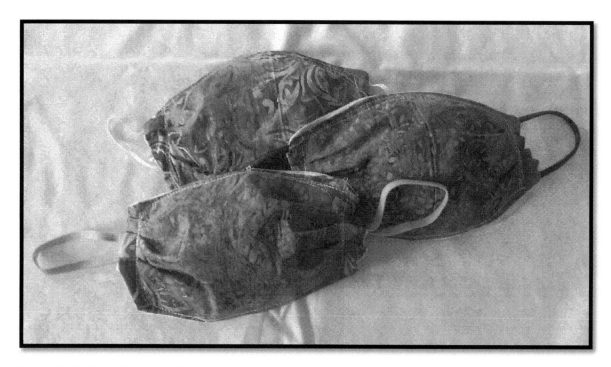

Figure 28 Masks made by Mary Zlotnick.

Mary Zlotnick[59], an artist in Brunswick County, was kind enough to make masks for the members of the Brunswick Search and Rescue team. Her efforts were most appreciated. She refused to take any payment for these stating that she just wanted to help. Others like her began the same quest. It was neighbors helping neighbors.

In the photograph of the masks above, note the back mask was made with elastic for the ear bands. Then, when elastic became unavailable, the maker switched to sewing binding tape. When that became unavailable, rubber bands had to suffice. Later ties were added instead of the ear bands, adapting to the availability of the materials.

---

[59] Mary Zlotnick. Web site: www.authenticpawleys.life.

Many others across the globe were making masks for their own families to use as they go to the grocery store, doctor, or other essential businesses. Anything from multiple

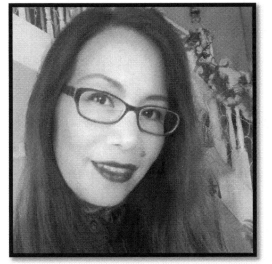

layers of cloth to cutting socks in a creative way making a non-sewn facial mask.

Many are sewing masks at home for friends and family and medical personnel finding themselves short of medical supplies. One such individual, Rema Juntoria Faircloth, of Varnamtown, North Carolina, made over a thousand masks for the children of the Philippines, her home country, after hearing of the shortage there. What a quiet hero, she continues to be.

Figure 29 Rema Faircloth Juntoria.

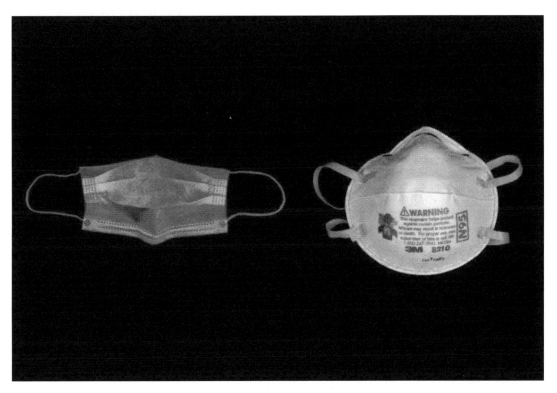

Figure 30 N95 Masks.

Figure 31 Christy Judah sports her puppy mask bandana.

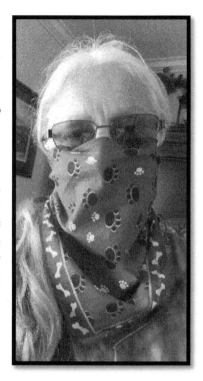

Facial coverings varied from official N95 masks to surgical and homemade masks, like the bandana.

Trying to purchase masks was a challenge for a while, especially for those who needed large quantities like hospitals and medical facilities. However, the earth's leaders were handling this, each for their own country. Masks later became quite plentiful whether handmade or produced and sold nearly everywhere. Every pattern, design imaginable and color came to the stores.

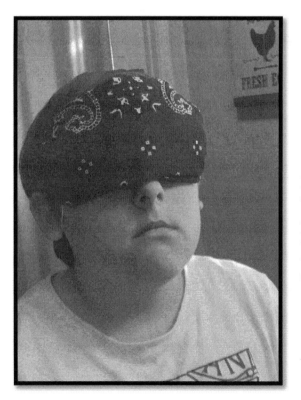

It is quite clear in the picture of Jacob Fisher that the children have their own take on the mask situation. Jacob Fisher was playing around with the first time he tries on a homemade *Rona Mask*/ aka bandana! Silly antics like this made us all smile during this scary time.

Figure 32 Jacob Fisher.

Then a month later, he is shown below with his mother, Jennifer Fisher, on their first outing wearing a handmade mask. Everyone debated diligently whether to leave the house but grocery shopping could not wait any longer.

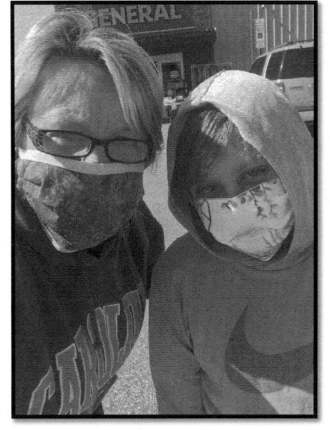

Figure 33 Jennifer Fisher and Jacob Fisher.

Stedman, NC.

On April 26th, 2021, while we can go out shopping and to restaurants here in North Carolina, masks are still the norm for most. Some are still anti-mask feeling the government either local or state or federal has no right to require us to wear masks, but when the state tells the business they may not open unless patrons wear masks, they have no choice but to require them to enter the store. Individuals still have the right to not enter if they feel strongly about the masks. Even some enter the store without masks and no one seems to say anything at this time. The author like many others, entering a business without a mask simply forgetting to grab it when leaving the car and like others, says, "Shoot, and marches right back to the car to get it." Better safe than sorry.

Volunteer Activities

In case you are wondering, yes, in the middle of this pandemic, volunteer fire departments, search teams and rescue squads continued to respond to requests for service. The Brunswick Search and Rescue Team, BSAR, North Carolina) was called to the site of a drowning where a terrible boat accident had happened. The team responded to help. Two died, two lived and one remained missing in the water. Six days later, members of the team responded to the Waccamaw River and met with the detectives and marine patrol units to search for the missing person. K9 Gibbs (handled by Christy Judah) indicated a likely location of the drowned person. After a large tree at that location was removed, the body was recovered. The family had their son to bury. Few were allowed to attend funerals and grieving often took place privately. While the COVID-19 disease ravaged the world, individual fire, rescue and emergency services continue to respond to the needs in the community across the nation as they do across the globe.

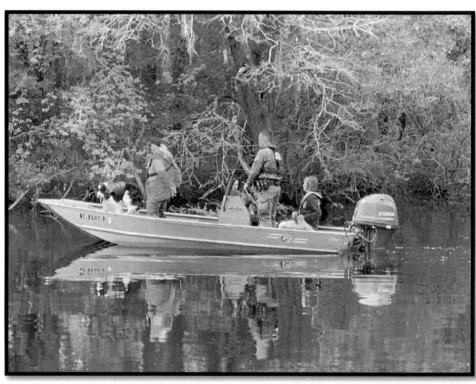

Figure 34 Brunswick Search & Rescue Team attempting to locate a drowned person.[60]

During early 2020, the members of Brunswick Search and Rescue were longing for the time they could get back into a regular training schedule and return to the woods and training grounds. The K9s were *antsy* and knew we were past due for a good day's training and a several day search. We thought that perhaps a little later this month we could do so. We were right.

Babies were still being born; families were still planning funerals both for natural deaths and the corona victims. Birthdays still come but the way of celebrating or mourning drastically changed; at least for now. Funerals and weddings were very private and small if held at all; birthday parties were practically non-existent. One family who defied the distancing guidelines held a birthday party with about 20 to 30 family members attending. Almost all of them got sick when one of the attendees, unknowingly carrying the virus but

---

[60] BSAR members Christy Judah, K9 Gibbs, Marci Anderson and Wildlife Officer on boat.

having no symptoms, infected most of those attending. One birthday guest died. The guilt that must be carried by those giving the party will probably last a lifetime. Bars, entertainment businesses, salons, and stores are closed except for grocery stores and pharmacies. For some reason, hardware stores are allowed to be open, so many shopped at Lowes or Home Depot to purchase needed supplies to spruce up the home and yard to pass the time. Most wore masks while shopping; few wore gloves. Only 100 patrons were allowed in the store at a time with specified entry and exit doors. A counter stood at the door giving one or two at a time permission to enter the store. This did help to maintain social distancing but seemed quite over the top to others.

Grocery Stores

Grocery stores were quite the experience. There were specially assigned times for the seniors to shop…the first hour of the day. Oh yah…we could be there by 7 am. Whoopie. This may mean we are safer not to be around the younger crowd who are not as apt to wear the PPE (personal protective equipment). The best part was most folks were wearing mask and many wearing latex gloves too. The sad part was everyone practically ignores everyone else, keeping their distance from each other and not even speaking; mostly. That eased up by March of 2021, thank goodness.

Certain aisles were totally empty or near about. It seems that once all this COVID information was distributed, some people hoarded very specific items…such as toilet paper. Before you knew it, those aisles were empty and shoppers were hoarding paper towels, napkins and anything else they could find to use for that personal purpose. When the grocery store manager was asked why we seemed to be so empty with that and some other products…he said that they have continued to get their regular order of groceries but they just disappear. Other items were not so easy to obtain, like rice or Duke's Mayonnaise. Not sure what the problem with the mayo was though. But all the southerners around North Carolina always pick Dukes over other brands.

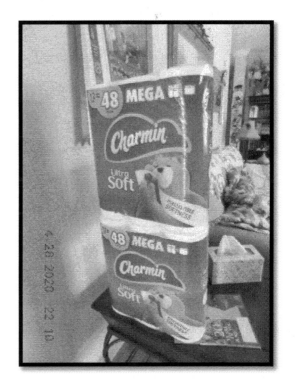

Figure 35 A scarce commodity…toilet paper.

Why would dish washing detergent be gone? "I actually had a friend who ordered this online today. Can you image having to order detergent online? I cannot really figure

131

out that one. There are lots of jokes going around about being out of a lot of items at the grocery store. The latest news is that I heard butter was hard to get. It is a good thing I bought two butters last trip."[61]

Like many stores which are allowed to be open (because they sell essential supplies and food), there is now a one-way IN and a one-way OUT with employees guarding the door. Notice the metal gates blocking entry through the regular doors in the photo below and the guard under the shelter to the left of the pictures.

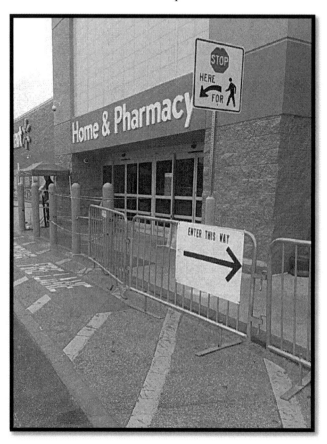

Figure 36 One Way Enter Sign.

Walmart…the store with everything you need, was open during the pandemic. It along with Home Depot and Lowes, and other like stores, were doing a brisk business. Some questioned why they can sell any product in the store when other, smaller businesses, deemed nonessential, had to remain closed as of April 23, 2020.

Once inside, many stores were limiting the number of customers allowed inside at one time, the aisles are labeled one-way traffic. Like many stores, there are now one-way

---

[61] Christy Judah.

aisles. "I got stuck in one today as they were stocking shelves at the other end and had to turn around and to back down a one-way aisle the wrong way. The looks I got when someone else entered that aisle was likely intended to convey to me, 'You are walking down the aisle the wrong way lady…pay attention.'

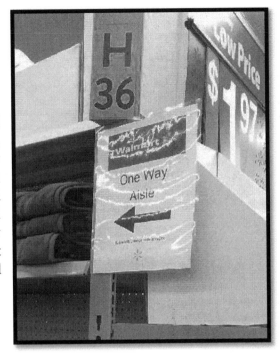

Figure 37 One-way aisle sign in Walmart.

Customers were pleased to see cashiers and other employees wearing masks and gloves, especially at restaurants. But the heart was heavy and anxious when handling money and goods in the stores. Many used a credit card so they would not have to touch the keypad of the debit card machine; or paid exact cash so as not to get any change returned. Many returned to their car, got out the antibacterial wipe or liquid and sterilized their hands before reaching for the steering wheel.

Paranoid or smart, who knows."[62]

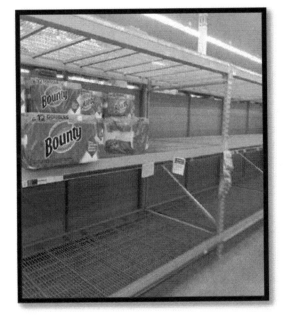

Figure 38 Paper goods shelves at Walmart, Shallotte, NC.

Paper goods were a valued commodity and surprisingly on the day this photo was taken a few packages of paper towels were available. No toilet tissue could be found. This was quite the topic of conversation throughout communities with everyone trying to figure out when the truck delivers to Food Lion or Piggly Wiggly.

---

[62] IBID.

Veterinarians

Even veterinarians and clinics have changed their methods of operation. The Brunswick Animal Hospital, like many others, required the customer to call-in upon arrival but remain in the vehicle. If it is necessary to bring the dog into the clinic, an employee would come to the car to pick up the animal. This helped to protect the employees, doctors, and clients. "Identifying myself as parked in spot #12, an employee picked up my dog; returned him in about ten minutes, and then brought me my pet's medication after a brief phone conversation with the vet. I then wrote a check, at the table set up outside of the clinic, wondering how long this practice would continue. It continues on as of March 21, 2021." By June 2021, one could finally go into the clinic, after calling to let them know you were in the parking lot and space was available in the waiting room. This after waiting a month for the appointment to arrive for a simple rabies shot. Man oh man.

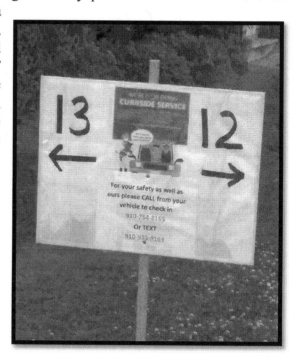

Figure 39
Vet Sign.

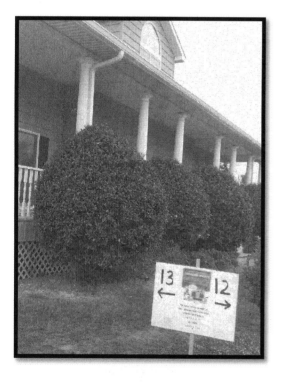

Figure 40 Brunswick Animal Hospital, Supply, NC.

Pets and Carol Sanner

Families continued to lose their loved ones with the added difficulty of holding a funeral since everyone was on lockdown. Persons were not allowed to meet in groups of more than ten; and depending upon where you live, groups of five. So, the generational tributes of the dead are either postponed or celebrated with few attending.

At the same time, the loss of a pet added to the stress of the time. Normally hugs are given and plenty of support is given by friends and family. This time losing a partner meant handling the pain alone. Carol Sanner, a search and rescue dog handler, described her personal situation on April 18th:

"A Humble Tribute to K9 Meg, 2005-2020"[63]

On April 18, 2020, we said goodbye to K9 Meg, age 15. The runt, but feistiest of a litter of 8 Border Collies from Washington State, she deserves tribute for her long and varied career as a working search dog.

Meg was trained as a SAR dog from the age of 8 weeks in Alaska and was certified in Wilderness Air Scenting by the age of 2. Unlike most search dogs, Meg was cross trained in Avalanche, Wilderness, Disaster, and Land Cadaver Search. She worked or trained in 10 states and formally logged over 3,000 hours of training. She rode in planes, helicopters, snow cats, snowmobiles, ATV's, boats, kayaks and scaled mountains in her missions and training. She performed her last multiday missing person search at the age of 13.

Meg's most notable mission was the recovery of a snowmobiler who perished in an avalanche in 2010. Over the course of a week's search- which had been suspended at one point for severe weather- the area had been combed by 160 volunteers and other K9 teams. On what was to be the last day of the organized search by Alaska State Troopers, Meg and I were flown on a helicopter to the remote incident site, about 60 miles south of Anchorage. Within 15 minutes of landing, Meg alerted on a single avalanche probe hole in the search area about the size of a football field. Subsequent probing by the search team near that spot revealed the body of the victim buried over 10 feet deep and about 12 feet from the probe hole.

Awaiting the recovery efforts, Meg spontaneously visited each of the 20 or so other searchers who had been stood down at the helicopter landing zone. Many were friends and colleagues of the victim. It gave great comfort and closure to family and searchers alike to know he was found at last. Meg was later warmly greeted by the hundreds who attended the victim's memorial. Every anniversary since, his family sent a package of treats and toys in gratitude for Meg's role in bringing him home.

---

[63] Carol Sanner. April 2020.

In 2014, Meg represented Deschutes County as one of 132 K9 teams from across the nation who was deployed to the tragic scene of the Oso, Washington mudslide that claimed the lives of 43 residents. Dogs were the key in locating remains buried up to 10 feet deep in mud and debris across a 1 square mile area. The dogs endured hypothermia, dehydration and were subjected to hazardous materials and then decontamination at the end of each shift. Yet there were no serious K9 injuries or after effects. All of the missing people were ultimately, found.

As a member of Deschutes County Search and Rescue Team from 2012 to 2018, K9 Meg and handler Carol helped revitalize the K9 unit and participated in 25 missions in 7 Oregon counties on behalf of the Deschutes County Sheriff's Office. In addition, Meg served as a DCSAR ambassador to countless public events and community outdoor education programs, conveying messages of backcountry safety and demonstrating how SAR dogs are utilized in a lost or missing person search.

From the handler's point of view, "Meg was a dog that comes along once in a handler's career. Stubborn, independent and relentless in play or work, she had all the best qualities of a search dog. Affectionate to those who needed her to be, but all business for me, her working partner; who was often little more than a delivery mechanism for a tennis ball or Frisbee to Meg.

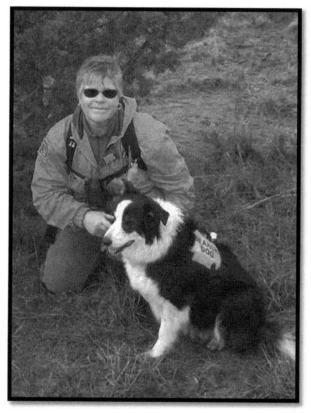

Play was work and vice versa. Her sassy disposition will be missed by all those who knew her. She greeted all her human friends with a tail wag and toy to throw. She brought joy to children in her search demonstrations, and comforted dementia sufferers in her visits to memory care homes."

Figure 93 Search & Rescue dog, Meg and Carol Jo Sanner April 18, 2020.

"Well, Meg, my friend and working partner, I was privileged to know you. This will be the last entry in your training log. Your work is done now. "Good girl, that'll do."

Animals as Carriers of the COVID-19 Virus - 2020

Earlier this year, the word was that people could not get it from animals and vice versa. Later, it became suspected that bats were the carrier and we could get it from food from the wet markets, who sold bats. Then that was disputed and it is supposed that it has come through the viral lab in Wuhan.

Then, a tiger in a United States zoo, contracted the virus. Then two, then three; supposedly getting it from either each other or a care taker at the zoo. Now, as of April 30th, it is known that we as humans can give the virus to the dog. More information on this will be forthcoming, for sure.

By April 30th, the CDC recommended that "Pet owners who contract COVID-19 should isolate themselves from their pets and other animals, and if possible, have another member of the household, a friend or neighbor care for the animal until they have recovered. Infected owners who cannot find another person to care for their animal should isolate themselves from the animal and should not pet, snuggle, kiss, share food or bedding with their pet."

The CDC continued to say that, "If a pet owner has contracted COVID-19 and has been in close contact with their pet and the animal starts to show signs of illness, the CDC warns against taking the animal to a veterinary clinic and instead recommends setting up a telemedicine consultation to determine next steps." They recommend that if a pet comes into contact with an infected human, owners should wash the coat well to remove the virus. Owners are advised to stock up with as two-week supply of food and medications just in case they contract it. When teleconferencing, they are advised to have their medical records handy, list of medications, and vaccination record. Symptoms may occur anywhere from 2 to 14 days after exposure just like in a human. Lordy, lordy.

The American Veterinary Medical Association

"To date, globally, the only pets incidentally exposed to COVID-19 that have tested positive, with confirmation, for SARS-CoV-2 are two pet dogs and a pet cat in Hong Kong, and two pet cats in the United States. The two pet cats in the United States both had signs of mild respiratory illness and were expected to make a full recovery. The pet cat in Hong Kong did not exhibit clinical signs of disease. Another pet cat in Belgium tested positive, but details around that case was less clear. The dogs and cats in Hong Kong were each in the care of and had close contact with a person who had been confirmed to have COVID-19. In the case of the cat in Belgium, other diseases and conditions that could have caused those same signs of illness were not ruled out and there are also questions about how samples demonstrating the presence of SARS-CoV-2 were collected and evaluated. That cat recovered," said the American Veterinary Medical Association.

The AMVA went on to publish on their web site that, "Until more is known about this virus, if you are ill with COVID-19 you should restrict contact with pets and other animals, just as you would restrict your contact with other people. When possible, have another member of your household or business care for any animals, including pets while you are sick. If you have a service animal or you must care for your animals, including pets, wear a cloth face covering; don't pet, share food, kiss, or hug them; and wash your hands before and after any contact with your pet, service animal, or other animals. You should not share dishes, drinking glasses, cups, eating utensils, towels, or bedding with other people or pets in your home."

Christy Judah, April 17th, 2020

Many folks took the stay at home orders as a good time to get caught up on home repairs, house cleaning and generally getting things done that have been on the list for quite some time. While on the stay-at-home order, my brother, Jamie Faircloth and his wife Rema, have helped to repair and fix up many things around my home during this lockdown time. The deck and kennels have a few new posts, and beautiful decorative lattice work was installed around the deck. The goldfish pond now has as working pump; all the weeds had to go and Rema and I worked hard to get it looking good. There is a new roof on the small storage room and it is nicely repainted. Despite all that exercise, I have probably gained a few pounds; not unlike many others stuck at home.

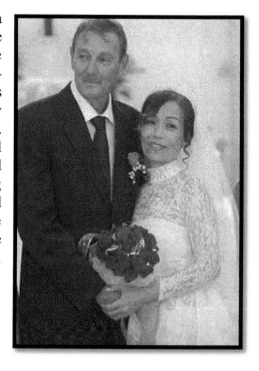

Figure 41 James and Rema Juntoria Faircloth.

"I do declare that I am not the only one who has put on a few pounds in the past several months. Others on Facebook have posted the same many times posting pictures of their yummy dishes. I just hate that the bakery down in Southport at the corner of Fish Factory Road is closed. Shawn Russell, author and friend, brought me a piece of strawberry cake baked by them. I was lucky enough to get a slice when she was here helping me deliver puppies the end of March. It was absolutely the best cake I have ever tasted. I am presently in wait for the day when I can visit them and buy one of those strawberry cakes for myself, my mom and dad and brother and sister-in-law."[64]

I would be remiss if I did not mention a common emotional status of others around me. Sometimes the nightmares come…drowning on a cruise ship. Or bugs all over me, and I cannot get them off. (However, this one may be rooted in too much watching television,

---

[64] Christy Judah.

especially *Naked and Afraid*.) In addition there is trouble sleeping and family squabbles getting blown out of proportion. There is a division among most people…the half which are afraid of the virus and trying their very best to follow the local, state and national guidelines. Then there are those who are having serious discussions about whether this is an illegal use of our government who seems to be controlling our every move. This is not unlike many citizens across the globe. Shall we be compliant and try our very best to get over this pandemic by following best practices or go about our activities with no masks or precautions. However, here in North Carolina, as of this date (April 30th), numbers continue to side with precaution; possibly because of increased testing but also because of localized spreading in nursing homes and businesses. Time will tell.

Zippy Cooper, Auburn, Georgia – April 18, 2020: Shown with her English Springer Spaniel, Yeager, International Champion Streamline Lenlear Sound Barrier.

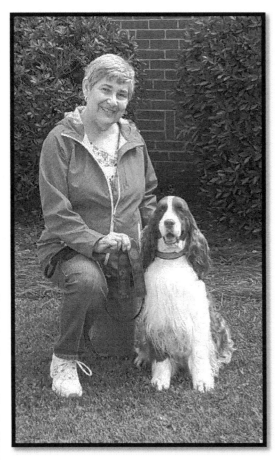

Figure 62 Zippy Cooper, GA.

Corona Confinement – The good, the bad and the very sad.[65]

"Confinement" is not only mandated by the authorities; it is also a state of mind. We can choose to be restricted or we can choose to simply refocus. I will always choose to refocus or be happy.

The Good that has come from my refocus is in several areas. I have more time to work with and train my dogs and my house is cleaner, but an unexpected benefit is that due to the travel restrictions, I have had to learn new technical ways to achieve my goals. In order to share in a birthday celebration for my daughter-In-law, I had to learn to do "Zoom" and in order to

---

[65] Zippy Cooper Essay. Corona Confinement – The good, the bad and the very sad. April 18, 2020.

get the groceries I wanted I used "Instacart" for the first time, and online Pizza delivery. I have a club meeting coming up and it will be conducted online.

Also, under the Good category, is that I have been motivated to give to others more than normal. I am not spending money on gas, dog classes, or eating out with friends, so there is a little extra to help someone else.

I am also very grateful for social media, like Facebook, in order to visit with friends, share photos, and yes, argue politics with strangers.

The Bad is that since I cannot go to my normal exercise class at the local YMCA, I have gotten fatter, stiffer and lazy. While there are exercise classes on U-tube, I can't seem to get motivated to participate.

The Sad is very sad. My dear cousin is in an Intensive Care Unit, on a ventilator, suffering from this COVID-19 virus. He is 70 years old and mentally challenged. They are trying a new experimental treatment on him, but his chances are not good. This is especially distressing since he doesn't understand what exactly is happening or why he is alone. The only comforting thing for me is that he is now in an induced coma and is no longer aware.

We, as a country, will get through this and in one way or another, we will be better people. Ronald Smith, of North Carolina, expressed his experiences which mirror so many others.

We Will Get Through This![66]   by Ronald Smith.

It's strange, when you hear a particular word, like smelling a certain aroma, your mind reaches into the billions of memories you have stored and retrieves one or two. This happened to me when the word "pandemic" began to appear in the media.

Having read the history of the 1918 flu pandemic that took the lives of some thirty million people around the world I thought about my grandmother. She hadn't been married all that many years and in 1918 was expecting her first child, my mother. She lived in the city in a neighborhood where the houses were relatively close together. I often wonder how concerned she was about what was going on in the rest of the world. Of course, she didn't have the "instant" communication sources we have today; just the local paper and the radio.

I wish I had talked to her about it, but growing up I was pretty ignorant on that subject. I remember she and my parents tell more tales about rationing during World War II than most anything else. Being a "baby boomer" I've seen my share of world altering events but never thought a pandemic would be one of them.

---

[66] Essay by Ronald Smith. April 2020.

I remember in the '50's when Polio made the headlines. The evening news on the television (black and white of course) ran stories on children and some adults who were confined to "iron lungs" and would be that way as long as they lived. I never knew anyone who had Polio. But I do remember taking the serum coated sugar cube at school that would safeguard me from this deadly disease.

I don't remember if our parents had to sign a consent form for us to be vaccinated or not. Just line up and be handed the cube and put it in your mouth and let it melt as you headed back to class. I remember getting shots for other things like typhoid and tetanus, and at Navy boot camp we got shots for who knows what and they were administered all at once with one of those "guns" that shot everything through your skin.

Then came Swine Flu, and, where I lived, we went to the local fire station and got a shot for that. When Hepatitis "B" was all the talk a series of three shots spread out over several months was on my agenda. A few years ago, I was advised (as I am now classified a senior) to get the pneumonia shot, which I did, and I am sure I had pneumonia shortly afterward!

Every fall it's the flu shot. And since I am more senior than I used to be, I now get the "super" flu shot designed for members of the older generation, myself included.

Now everything has changed. With the exception of the few people over 102 years old, we are all dealing with something we have never experienced before and never thought we would be given all the advances in science we have seen during our lifetime.

Everyone is handling this situation in their own way. I'm involved in a lot of "stuff" and right now I can't do the things that occupied a lot of my time. As chairman of the town's Planning Commission, my meetings have been cancelled and projects envisioned by the town are on hold for the time being.

I play in a band. We do what I call the "retirement home circuit" as we play music at various facilities around the area that are primarily for the many that need assisted living care. These folks don't get out much, so, my band brings music they are familiar with to them once a month and we do it for free as our way of giving back to the community. I always enjoy seeing the smiles on the faces of those we play for. That's not happening right now.

My Lions Club is not meeting. While our club is small, we do a lot for the community. That's not happening right now. I volunteer at the elementary school and read with third graders once a week. Schools are closed. I'm not reading with anyone right now.

I enjoy my church. Our minister is really good and well liked. It's a small congregation so everyone knows everyone. Nobody is going to church right now. Saturdays I am usually at the Farmers Market visiting with my friends. While you can contact your favorite vendor and pick up your order, Farmers Market in its usual form is not happening right now.

I am on the ballot for the next town election, hoping to be the next mayor. Even though I know a lot of the people who live in this small town of five hundred, I had planned on trying to visit as many voters as possible and meet those I don't know. Not going to happen.

So, what am I doing during this time of insulating and isolating oneself from others? I am staying home as much as possible. I only go to the post office a couple of times a week rather than every day as I used to do. I only go to the grocery when necessary. At least the bank, my only other stop, is drive-in window only so I can go there, but I miss going inside and seeing my friends who work there.

I have a small business where I quilt for people. No customers, no income from that. I work part-time at the local funeral home. I've been a funeral director for forty-five years, but right now no funerals, mostly cremations, no income from that. I write articles for the local monthly paper. Since the paper generates its income from advertisements, and everything has been closed or cancelled, the paper is "on hold" for the foreseeable future. No income from that.

Being a "senior" does have its advantages. I receive Social Security so I still have an income. And I can take comfort that my children, all grown, are in professions that are deemed "essential" and are pretty certain they will not lose their jobs.

I am keeping busy. There are always things to do around the house and lots of grass to cut. Even though I live in town, I have over eight acres to cut and mow. And I am still writing articles so I will be ready when the paper comes back to life.

What has really concerned me the most about this pandemic is how people are reacting to stay at home orders and safe distancing? When I make those necessary trips out and see people with no face mask, no gloves, with obviously no sense of the seriousness of this matter, I just can't fathom their ignorance. And to have some people still think it is not all that bad or a conspiracy of some kind when, as I write this, over 55,000 have died and a "good day" in New York is when only five hundred people die, makes me wonder if we have bred a bunch of people with no common sense? I just don't understand.

I still think about my grandmother. But I also think about my grandchildren. I won't be telling them about my pandemic experience because they are living through this time also. They will have their own stories for their children and grandchildren. So here is what I'm going to do. I will continue to go out only when necessary and only to places that are necessary. I will continue to wear my mask and gloves, carry my hand sanitizer, and wash my hands a lot. I will learn some new songs so when the band can play together again, I will be ready. And, when I say my prayers at night, I will continue to ask God to be with those who are suffering from this pandemic, help us to get through this situation we find ourselves in, and to keep me and my family safe.

I know we will get through this. And when you see me and I have my mask on, just remember that behind the mask is a smile because I am glad to see you.

Jobs and Unemployment

Many are unemployed at the highest rate from any time in the past. Students lost jobs at closed colleges, and most businesses were closed unless designated as essential. The federal government, under President Trumps' leadership, designated funds for elevated unemployment benefits for those who qualify, and in essence doubled the normal unemployment check amount. As of April, the 18th, 2020 many awaited those checks. This tentatively would later play into a labor force need with some not wanting to go back to work being able to make more on unemployment than employment.

As of April 30th, 2020, "Americans filed 3.8 million new jobless claims last week, the Labor Department reported Thursday, pushing the six-week claims tally to 30.3 million as the coronavirus pandemic battered the economy."[67]

"The new report, which covers the week ending April 25, likely understated the total number of Americans who lost their jobs as the death toll from the disease climbed above that of the Vietnam War."[68]

Small business owners had the opportunity to apply for small business loans which if used for personnel salaries, were not payable back to the federal government. However, news interviewing may owners claim that the cost of re-opening and restocking (especially with items which expire like food products or such, will take so many thousands of dollars that it is fruitless to pay the employees while they are furloughed because they cannot afford to open back up when all the closings are lifted. A vicious circle was how some described the shut-down of American businesses.

A beauty salon owner in Georgia, disobeyed the close order for salons and personal care businesses and opened her business the week of May 9th. She was arrested and sent to jail. When she came in front of the judge the next day, she calmly explained that her stylists and she had children to feed and no income coming in. She had no choice but to open so she could feed her children. The judge dismissed the charges and released her and the salon has stayed open. The whole country watched as this drama unfolded on television.

Restaurants

Restaurants closed their doors and provided food for pick-up only. This, of course, put many at risk of not having a business to open up when all the restrictions are lifted as most have much less income than pre-COVID-19.

---

[67] Politico. By Rebecca Rainey. Coronavirus-driven unemployment claims surpass 30 million. April 30, 2020. https://news.yahoo.com/labor-department-reports-3-8-123115233.html.
[68] IBID.

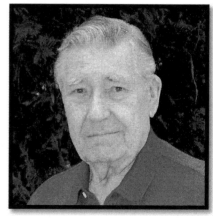

Figure 66 Photographer John Muuss.

John Muuss, of St. James, NC, said, "When COVID-19 hit and we observed the world around us rapidly changing, we changed our thinking too. The members of the Richard H. Stewart, Jr., Saint James American Legion Post 543 began asking what we could do to help those who had helped our veterans across Brunswick County throughout the years. One area being hit the hardest was our small business restaurants, and more specifically the servers who work there. Being paid as little as $2.13 per hour while the balance is being made up through tips. These workers were largely unable to benefit from the Payroll Protection Plan.

The Post recently supported one such Southport establishment by setting up a special night to help servers and getting the world out across the area. Members of Post 543 served as volunteers guiding traffic and running orders from the wait staff inside to the waiting customers who remained inside their vehicles. The outpouring of support by our Brunswick County family was deeply moving and appreciated by the employees."[69] Similar events are taking place all across our county supporting the restaurants and employees.

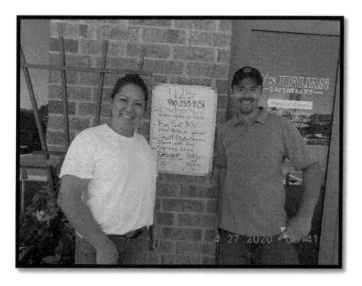

All restaurants are now closed (April 28, 2020) and serving only take-out orders. From McDonalds to Pizza Parlors, and fancy cloth napkin restaurants, everyone is either closed or offering take-out.

Figure 42 M'Ds Italian Restaurant Owner and employee; Diane Kingsbury, owner, and Josh Boggess, server.

---

[69] John Muuss. Certified Professional Photographer. Town of St. James, NC. johnmuuss@gmail.com

In Bolivia, NC, *D's Italian Restaurant,* posted some items to order in anticipation of the day they can open again. Still serving take-out, they are thankful for the business they *are* getting.

The Oriental restaurant is in the same shape in the same shopping center off of highway 211 in Brunswick County, NC. The following sign was posted on their door and read: *The door is lock. Call 910-XXX-XXXX to ask if your food is ready. Please keep 6 feet apart from each other. Sorry for the inconvenience.*

This restaurant, *Wok & Roll,* even built a semi-safe *slide through opening* in his business as a safety precaution. This restaurant is located in a shopping center off of Highway 211 in Bolivia, NC. Stay outside to order and receive your food. Pass payment through slit but pick up your eating utensils in an open-air box on the table outside. Hummmm….

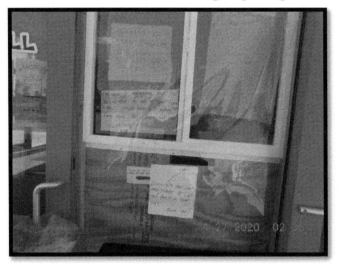

Figure 43 Wok & Roll Restaurant.

Figure 44 Wok & Roll.

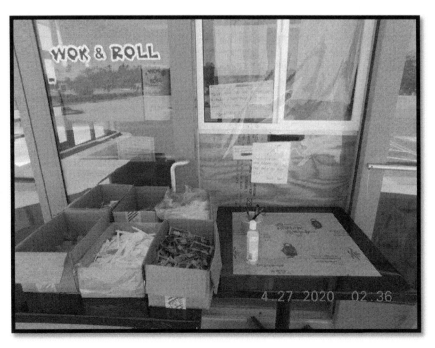

The *Wok & Roll* also placed their condiments, plastic ware, etc., on a table outside for customers to help themselves.

Other restaurants posted that they are open and serving take-out only. By May 11, 2020 some ice cream shops were open, but only allowing a few folks in at a time so they can pick out their ice cream flavor for their cone or sundae. No eating was allowed inside, and tape covered the outdoor picnic table prohibiting anyone from sitting. So, the patrons stand next to their vehicle in the parking lot to enjoy the treat. Such is how it was at *Beaches and Cream Ice Cream Shop* in Holden Beach, North Carolina in May of 2020. Patrons look forward to the time when the heat arrives this summer that they can sit down inside to enjoy their cone.

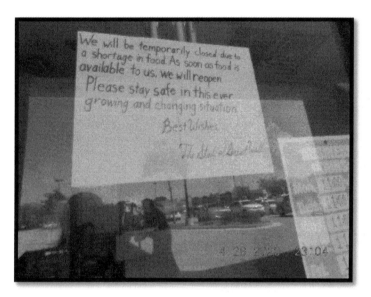

The Great Wall Oriental restaurant in the Food Lion shopping center in Holden Beach, NC posted a sign on their door indicating a **shortage of food**; and will reopen when the situation changes. It is unclear why there was a shortage of food…only supposition would answer that question at this time.

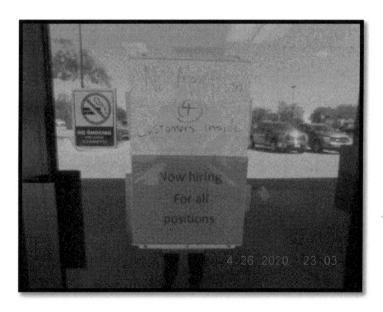

Restaurants like the *Surfer Café*, allowed only four customers inside at a time to order their take-out; and were *hiring for all positions.*

146

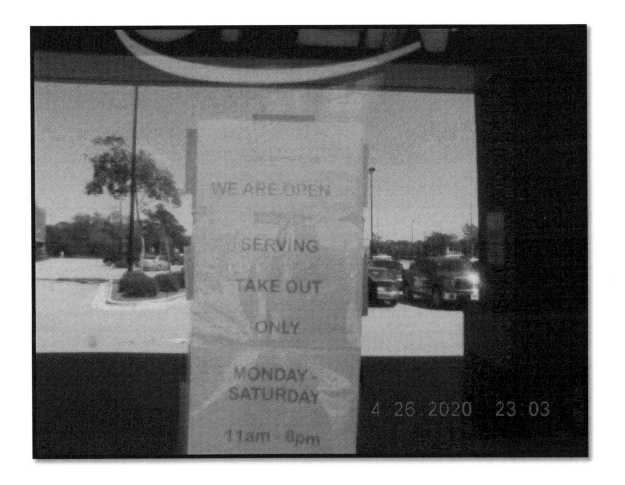

Figure 45 Restaurant sign; No more than 4 customers inside.

In other businesses, local musicians, Tom Yandle, Paul Kumlin, and Willis Alston continued to visit McDonalds fast food restaurant in Shallotte, NC, *inside,* regularly, to play their guitars and ukuleles; and sing out the old 1940s and 50s songs to the delight of patrons; despite the Covid restrictions; probably not mentioned in the governors' guidelines. Yodeling is not dead yet in rural communities of the south.

April 18th, 2020 – U.S. Air Force Academy Graduation[70]

Vice- President Mike Pence spoke to the graduates of the 2020 U. S. Air Force Academy, in Colorado Springs, Colorado. Their graduation ceremonies were minus the families of the cadets because of the time in which we live but we all know that they could not be any prouder of these men and women. They sat with six feet between chairs on the athletic fields and looked so smart in their white pants, gold waistband sashes, caps and blue jackets.

Mr. Pence told them, "Some graduates will become our next astronauts, pilots and commanders. Many come from parents who had also attended the US Air Force Academy. These fine officers will serve our country well." Vice President Pence reminded them all "You are an inspiration to all." With the flag of the United States flying behind him, he told them that, "Americans will protect the most vulnerable and heal our land. Now comes your time to do yours, defending the people of this nation. Long after the virus is defeated your mission will go on. On behalf of the Commander-in-chief in these challenging times, I admonish you to be vigilant, respect the chain of command, and take care of each other and all of those who report to you. Every decision you make matters to the security of this nation. Lead yourself first and be men and women of integrity. Be diligent to cultivate these virtues and you will lead those airmen with great distinction. The American people are counting on you."

"Today is a special day for you and the American Air Power…on this day in 1942 after the attack on Pearl Harbor, not just a day that lived in infamy but a day that shocked the nation and pulled us into war. Lt. Jimmy Dolittle led an air attack 668 miles away and that mission inspired the nation and gave the American people confidence that we would prevail. I believe with all my heart, from Americans looking around the country, and seeing you brave men and women, setting you off on your mission, you will also inspire confidence that we will prevail against the invisible enemy as well. Many heroes have passed through these halls that have defended freedom in their time like you will in your time."

He continued by saying, "As you take to the air you will go with the confidence of the Command-in-Chief and the confidence of the American people. And He who brought you this far will never forsake you. His right hand will hold you fast. Congratulations to the Air Force Academy of 2020 in the United States Air Force and the United States Space Force. God bless our Air Force and our Space Force and God bless the United States of America."

---

[70] Notes from the speech given by Vice President Mike Pence on April 18th to the graduates of the U.S. Air force Academy in Colorado Springers, Colorado.

⁷¹
Update to the Cadets from the US Air Force Academy Superintendent on March 6, 2020

The USAFA,

"This is our new "normal" (or, I haven't left USAFA since March 6th!). We are going to be in this condition for a while, so start planning and adapting. As an Air Force, we should not expect a distributed vaccine or return to pre-COVID operations until possibly the summer of 2021, if not longer. My call to Team USAFA: be creative, be deliberate! Be innovative in the management of our workplaces, blue/silver teaming, etc. We need long-term solutions to these restrictions. Establishing consistent, sustainable practices in this new environment is crucial to our morale, health, and continued mission success. If you are expecting a date that we will get back to normal, you will be disappointed. Posture yourselves and your teams as if these are permanent changes, said Superintendent Lt. General Jay B. Silveria. (Lieutenant General; fighter pilot; Deputy Commander, U.S. Air Forces Central Command; Commander, U.S. Air Force Warfare Center; Vice Commander, 14th Air Force; aide-de-camp to Supreme Allied Commander Europe.)

He continued in his weekly update telling the cadets, "Further, as we work through the change in our working condition – communicate, communicate! At times, it may feel like over-communication but the environment we are working in now requires us to err toward that side of spectrum. If you are experiencing an issue that impacts you, it likely has an impact on your team and even others across the installation."

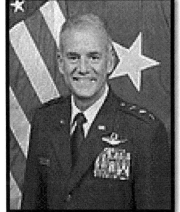

Figure 46 Lt. Gen. Jay B. Silveria.⁷²

The Academy, like many other schools, universities and other educational institutions, modified their instructional models by using TEAMS and Zoom...computer meet-up programs. Lt. General said, "Conditions can change so we will all need to remain flexible... that it is our goal to bring the Cadet Wing back to the Colorado Springs area for class in August. The process to bring everyone back and what that looks like is still being developed. The most important point for now is that everyone needs to set realistic expectations about what USAFA will be like in the fall because it will not be the USAFA we all knew when we dispersed around the

---

⁷¹ USAFA Superintendent Weekly Update on March 6, 2020. https://www.usafa.edu/app/uploads/Supt-Weekly-Update-7.pdf.
⁷² Jay B. Silveria. Photo from Wikipedia. https://en.wikipedia.org/wiki/List_of_superintendents_of_the_United_States_Air_Force_Academy.

country or to our homes for teleworking." He charged the cadets to, "Be good examples in your local community. The rules and policies on the installation may differ slightly from those of the state, but when we are off-duty, we are all residents of Colorado. Consider that each interaction you have increases the risk to our mission."

Lt. General Silveria shared that:

•On Wednesday 6 May, those that have installation access can come on base to fish and hike and bike the trails. We are comfortable we can do this safely as these activities occur outdoors and we can maintain social distancing.

• Also, on the 6th of May the North Gate will open from 0600-0800 and again from 1500 to 1700.

• With the extension of the Stop Movement Order by SECDEF, the intent remains to minimize travel. For military members, leave is still limited to a 100-mile radius of USAFA.

"He continued by saying, "We need Team USAFA to stay healthy and mitigate risk to the maximum extent. Internalize that any risks you take, risk the USAFA family and they risk the mission. We are all in this together – please look out for each other. Look out for your teammates at USAFA; look out for the folks in your community. Stay healthy, stay connected." Thanks, JS.

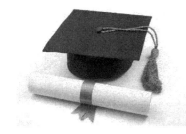

High School Graduation and Public School Education

With the virtual lock-downs and closing of schools in all states, seniors in high school did not get to look forward to walking across the stage and accepting their diplomas this year, (2020). Some ended up being held in the spring of 2021 but not many. There were virtual graduation ceremonies without the graduates and their families. There were also virtual proms those years. It was a sad way to end a high school career.

At home with their children and providing home-schooling, parents and caregivers gained a new respect for teachers. One mother, who shall remain unnamed, had three children she was home-schooling. One was in elementary school, we shall call him E; one is in middle school, we shall call him J; and one in high school, called I. Both I and J were given assignments by their teachers using computer programs and additional teacher assigned activities. They were allowed to complete their assignment fairly independently.

E, a bit younger, was more of a challenge. Younger students were often given workbooks and written assignments much more often than while learning in the school building. This situation for a bright elementary student brought some unrest in this household learning environment. He did not understand and demanded answers to why he could not do his assignments on the computer. This caused the mother to put her child on in-school suspension several times already. E was advised to talk to the principal (his Dad) if he had any more questions about the assignment and manner in which his local officials and state government leaders decided he completes his assignments. Fourth grade can be tough. Of great interest was when his state would decide students could return to their regular schooling back in the classrooms of the old school building. With much patience his parents continued doing the very best they could as the governor announced on April 30th that the state school system will be closed for the remainder of the 2019-2020 school year and beyond. Finally, by the end of April 2021, his school reopened for in person learning four days a week. Students attended on Monday, Tuesday, Thursday and Friday with Wednesday reserved for cleaning. This was the schedule in one particular school system; each decided when they would re-open according to state guidelines, and local statistics.

Around the nation, school systems provided students with equipment like laptops and technology; internet providers provided free internet; and everyone worked to provide a method to continue education for the students. The at home teachers, aka moms, did not appreciate a phone call from the principal of the real school to complain about the student…who happened to be sleeping at the computer while zoom classes were conducted. Oh me, fifth grade was tough too. Geez, how was a mom supposed to work at home and still provide all the supervision…one wondered how the moms who left their children alone at home fared.

Parents without any advanced education found these home assignments quite a challenge. Children with educational disabilities were probably the most difficult of all to monitor and educate. Those virtual learning environments provided challenges such as never before experienced by teachers or parents. Life continued; education or some semblance of it, did too.

It was heartwarming to hear stories of principals and teachers across the state and nation, who took their own time and effort to deliver graduation yard signs to each graduate of their senior class. Some even delivered them personally to the graduates trying to make their graduation a special time despite the fact that there were no graduation ceremonies.

On the other hand, many worry that the lack of in school education for the school year 20-21 will put an entire generation in trouble in the long run… especially for the learning disabled; falling further behind. Others believe we will get back to our normal educational practices and education will surely resume by the school year 2021-2022. The future will tell the story.

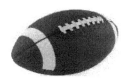

The National Football League and Other Sports

The National Football League opted to do virtual ceremonies of the draft in 2020. Videos connected coaches, and candidates for the draft to each other from living rooms and basements. The nation watched as one draft pick after another was selected for the new teams in the NFL. It is still unclear if football games in the U.S. will be attended by fans or recorded and only shown on television. Either way, fans are looking forward to getting back into their sports routines with their favorite team. All were hoping that football will go on as planned in August, September and beyond. That was not to happen. Fans were not allowed to come to the stadiums and TV broadcasts actually put pictures of fan in the seats in the stadium and supplemented with canned applause. Not really realistic but the best they could do. Some games were cancelled or postponed when too many of the players came down with COVID. What a season.

In the meantime, during April, all of the major speedway races were cancelled. Some golf and tennis events were still on the calendar for June and July and beyond others cancelled.

Sporting events will follow as the nation slowly re-opens. Sunday afternoon games will continue with a bit of a new twist...no fans in the stands. By June of 2021, the fans were back to most stadiums. Eventually we will get back to normal.

Figure 47 Holden Beach, NC.

Holden Beach, North Carolina on the first weekend that the beaches were re-opened.

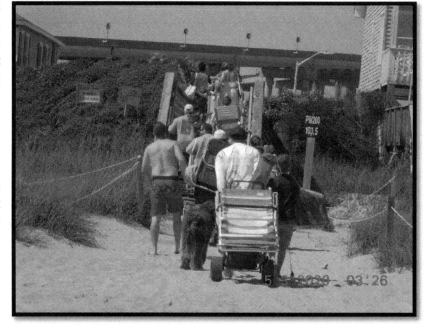

The Beaches

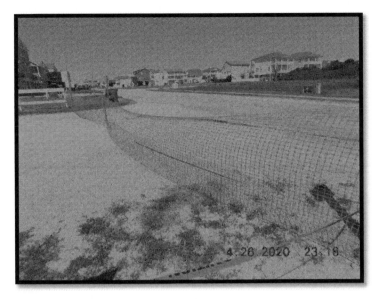

Oh, the beaches. When the beaches first closed, around the country, it was a huge topic of conversation all across coastal areas. From photographs of thousands of people on the beach, many appearing young, the regular spring break activities that college students have practiced for years seemed to continue. Most leaders were literally begging that younger crowd to leave the beaches despite most media who said that the teens and early twenty-something's were not as much at risk as those in older age or those with other contributing health issues.

Figure 48 Holden Beach netting.

Fencing at Holden Beach blocking parking in the public parking areas in March through May 3rd, 2020.

Later the science caught up and it is now known that this virus can affect us all.

In addition, the fear was that these young folks who could be carriers of the virus, and also be without symptoms, could infect many, if not hundreds or thousands more. Some listened. Some did not. Quite probably, they infected many in the coming weeks a numbers climbed. The beaches which had been re-opened in small steps, easing the guidelines, mostly by beach town governments themselves, found varying results.

At first, it seemed the beaches were closed to all. Then all public parking areas were taped off and the beaches were only open to those who actually lived on the beach, but mostly still requiring visitors to stay in very small groups of 5 or less. Plastic fencing was posted across all public parking in Holden Beach, NC, on April 28th, 2020, shown in the photograph above.

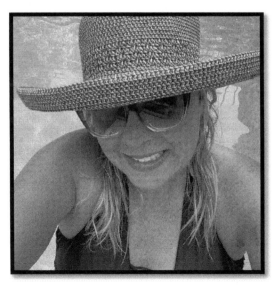

Figure 49 Jennifer Fisher.

153

"A few days ago, some of the beaches in Brunswick County were opened to those wanting to get exercise, but parking remained closed. Therefore, only those with friends who had homes on the island could park and walk on the beach. All public parking areas were closed. "This too shall pass," said General Douglas McArthur quite a few years ago but still relevant today.

Updates from April 30, 2020

At today's' teleconference briefing in Brunswick County, there were concerns expressed by the Health and Human Services director, David Stanley, about the way we open the beaches here in our county. (April 30, 2020.) Ocean Isle Beach was opened to the public with parking available. According to Mr. Stanley, the opening of our county, and specifically our beaches, needs to be a very thoughtful and careful plan based upon data. Opening the beaches should consider whether short term rentals will be allowed (as it was in Ocean Isle Beach) and take into consideration the increased traffic, increased law enforcement activity, reduced supplies which may affect our grocery stores and related businesses. He encouraged our local municipalities, like those around the nation, to base decisions on data keeping in mind that you will not see, most likely, immediate ramifications of these changes for two weeks, while non-symptomatic persons begin to infect others.

Those counties such as Horry County, South Carolina, just south of Brunswick County, opened their facilities the past few days. It is noted that they have a larger number of COVID cases than Brunswick as of this date: Over 200 to our 43. Many are worried Brunswick citizens will go south to shop and play, bringing the virus back here for an increase in our cases. We will know in about two weeks.

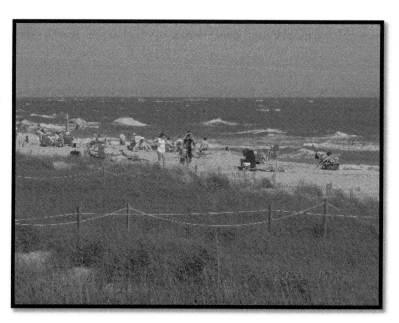

Figure 50 Beaches.

By May 5, 2020, Holden Beach had opened. Thousands flocked to the sandy beaches under perfect sunshine. However, time would tell if the crowds were safe or exposed to the virus during their respite.

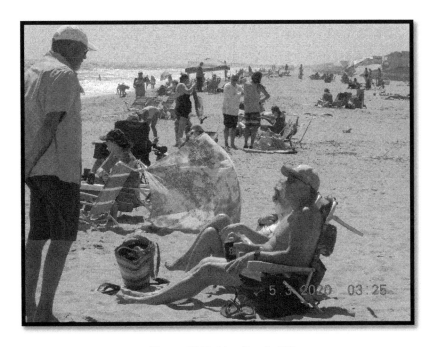

Figure 51 Holden Beach, NC.

Parking lots were so full (now opened) that premium parking became anywhere a patch of grass existed. A quick scan of the license plates showed most were North Carolina license plates. The weather cooperated and, in some ways, helped the occasion with sunshine eradicating some of the virus (hopefully) with UV rays. (Perhaps?)

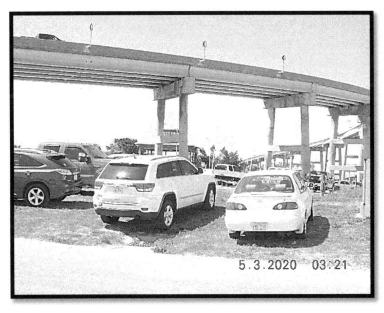

Figure 52 Holden Beach parking.

In California, when families flocked to the beaches in large numbers, the Governor responded by closing the beach back up. (April 30, 2020).[73] Starting that weekend, the coast would remain closed.

"Gov. Gavin Newsom is expected to announce that all California beaches and state parks will close in an unprecedented move to enforce the statewide shelter-in-place order and reduce the spread of coronavirus, according to a memo by the California Chiefs Association. The beach closures will go into effect at noon Friday, May 1, according to the memo that was sent to law enforcement agencies across the state."[74]

In Southport, North Carolina, even benches facing the water and marsh, were taped off and hoped to prohibit people from coming to relax on them.

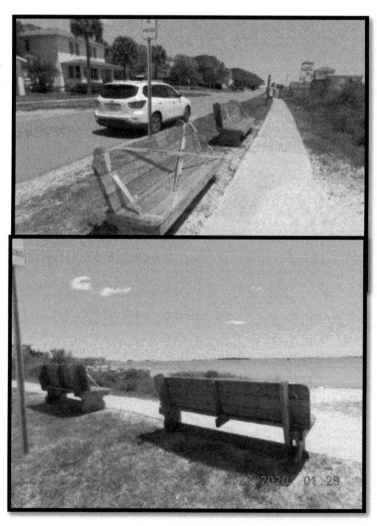

Figure 53 Southport Coast.

Many wondered if this *really*

made sense.

[73] All California beaches, state parks expected to close — including Pismo Beach
Sacramento Bee. Cassandra Garibay. Sacramento Bee. April 30, 2020.
[74] IBID.

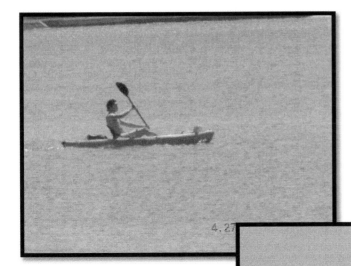

The bays are so close, yet so far away for a resident of Southport who wants to just sit and relax and watch the water. But nothing stopped this lone kayaker or shrimper.

Figure 54 Kayaker near Sunset Harbor, NC.

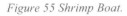

Figure 55 Shrimp Boat.

Figure 56 Pier entry ways are blocked.

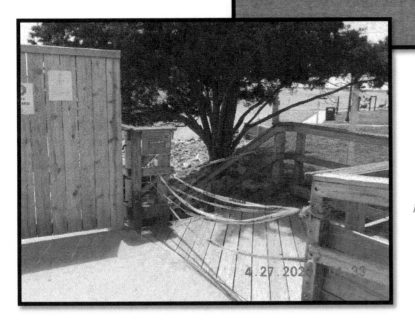

157

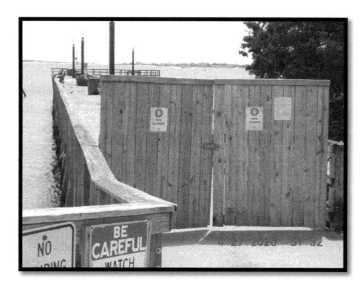

Figure 57 Southport, NC Pier.

So close to good fishing, yet so far away. A closed Southport, NC pier.

Figure 58 Small Town Police Department.

Figure 59 Police departments adapt.

Police departments implemented social distancing and closed offices referring visitors to call 9-1-1 if it was an emergency. Have no fear, as they were still on the job with their masks and gloves, working from home, and still arresting the criminals as needed.

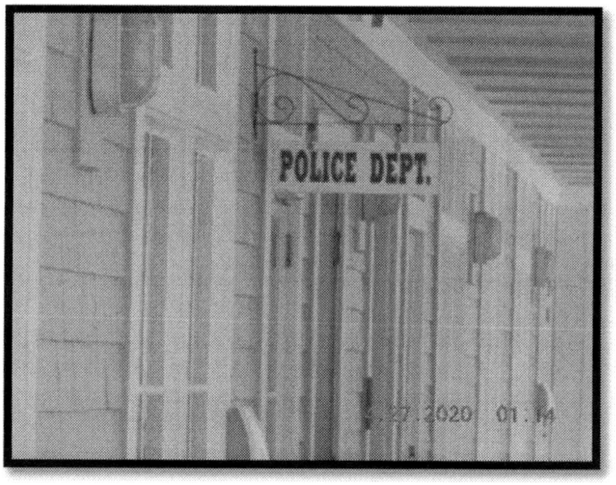

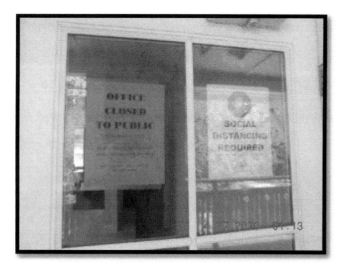

Police
Department Entry door.

Office Closed to Public.

Social Distancing Required.

158

Small Business Owners

Small business owners followed the guidelines and direction of their governors, national leaders and city officcials as they closed up shop.

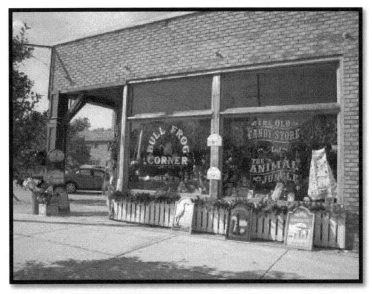

Figure 60 Bullfrog Corner.

Marianne and Ernie Long, owners and proprietors of *The* ***Bullfrog Corner*** (a very popular business in Southport, NC) holds a sign explaining that she is closed for now.

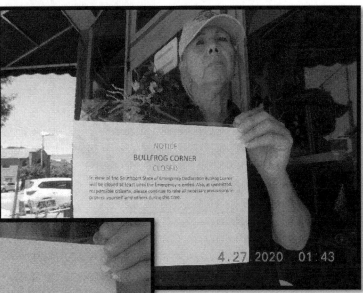

NOTICE
BULLFROG CORNER
CLOSED

In view of the Southport State of Emergency Declaration Bullfrog Corner will be closed at least until the Emergency is ended. Also, as committed, responsible citizens, please continue to take all necessary precautions to protect yourself and others during this time.

4.27.2020 01:43

Questions remained why some businesses were allowed to open and businesses such as the *Bullfrog Corner* were required to close.

Figure 61 Bullfrog Corner Closed.

"In view of the Southport State of Emergency Declaration, Bullfrog Corner will be closed at least until the emergency is ended. Also, as committed, responsible citizens, please continue to take all necessary precautions to protect yourself and others during this time." 2021 saw the *Bullfrog Corner* reopening to customers and back to the new normal. Many other small businesses were not as lucky and will not be re-opening. They had lost too much income during the year they were closed.

Swanson Realty

Realtors *were* allowed to operate with safety precautions and Tracy Swanson, of Swanson Realty, posted a sign on her office door saying that she is open and asks clients to call for an appointment.

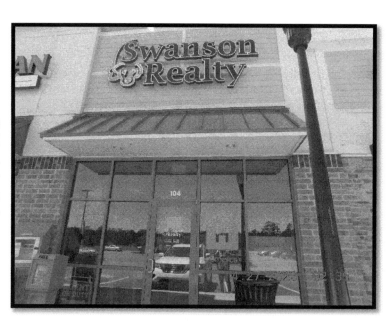

Figure 62 Swanson Realty, Bolivia, NC.

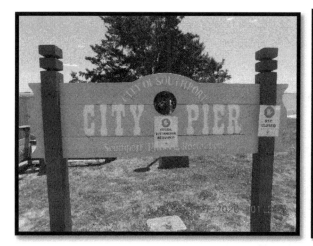

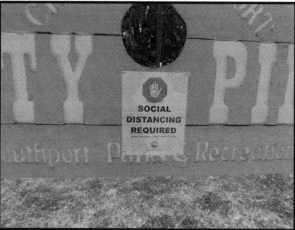

Figure 63 Southport City Pier.

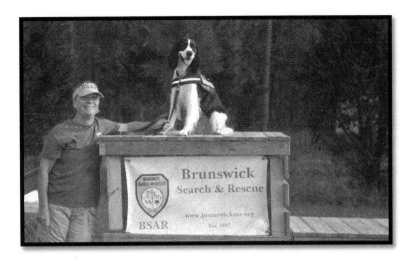

Marci Anderson Shares her Story

Marci Anderson, and her husband Brian, shared their experiences with this virus. Residing in Sneads Ferry, NC, Marci stated, "I am the polar opposite of a germaphobe. I have always operated under the assumption that the more I was exposed to germs, the less likely that I would get sick.

Enter COVID-19, Coronavirus, or as I have come to refer to it as, Rona. She blew into town and turned everything upside down. I was convinced initially that the hype was driven by social media; and the hysteria that grew did not change my opinion. However, it did not go away and when the lockdown came, with the guidance of social distancing, I started to see changes in my life that I did not like or appreciate."

"First there was the hoarding. I told myself it wasn't a big deal until I started running out of popular items like toilet paper and rice. One funny story about TP procurement had me slinking out of the Harris Teeter with a 24-pack like I had just robbed a bank," Anderson said.

"My best rice story was seeing some bulk bags of rice at the Turtle Hospital where I volunteer. Evidently, if turtles hitch a ride to warmer waters, they get rice filled socks micro-waved to warm them so that they don't get too cold on the ride. I have to admit I looked at those bulk bags and wondered whether I could talk them into letting me purchase one to get me through the quarantine," Anderson shared. She went on to say, "But, all in all, other than finding it amusing what folks were hoarding, I didn't have a terrible time getting by with what was stocked at our local grocery store. We did stock up prior to the stay at home order, so going to the grocery store was not necessary as often as I had gone in the past. It was still an adventure every single time."

She went on to share that, "I did not feel like going to the store could expose me to the virus that would most definitely kill me should I contract it (if you listened to the new.) I did start putting together my end of life documents as if I was currently on a respirator with no chance of surviving. I hated what I was becoming but there wasn't anything I could do except follow the guidance provided and choose the right course of action for me. The hardest part was not being able to visit my Dad who lives in a memory care facility which was locked down tight. They did manage to do one Facebook chat and then got Zoom so we could have a weekly family video call and I think that helped all of us. I understand (kind of) the need to lock down those facilities but it doesn't make it any easier to be apart from my Dad. I miss going to see him."

Anderson continued by saying, "I also miss my sister who has Multiple Sclerosis (MS) and whom I would put in the vulnerable category. I go over to her house and talk to her, keeping a safe distance, in the garage. Stupidly, really, since I would bring her some item that she had asked for which, according to the pundits, could have the virus on it; and then it could transfer to her if she touched the item and then touched her eyes, nose, or mouth." She continued by saying, "I miss being able to go to the Seaview Pier for breakfast every once in a while. I miss being able to go into a store without slinking around and worrying that I am going to contract the virus. I miss being able to purchase all those many items that were hoarded early on. I miss being able to go to training with my colleagues on the Brunswick Search and Rescue. But this will all be over eventually and we will resume some type of normal."

Moving from State to State: 2020 --The year of Tragedies and Blessings

By Jeanne Haynes, Mebane, NC   3/31/2021

As the COVID-19 Pandemic began storming across the world in the fall of 2019, I was in full swing of starting a new chapter in my life at the young age of 72. After 18 years of living in Wilmington, NC (rated as one of the best retirement beach towns in NC), I had decided to move closer to my daughter in Chapel Hill, NC. After all, family and pets are the most important part of one's life. Wilmington had provided me with a fully active retirement lifestyle including: a part-time job at New Hanover Regional Hospital in the HR department, serving on multiple committees in church and other organizations, while enjoying many social groups. Wilmington's many cultural venues were always interesting and I was living in my dream retirement townhome.

My expectations were to immediately transfer my current retirement lifestyle to my new home. This train of thought stopped abruptly in March of 2020 when we learned how COVID-19, the world-wide pandemic, was changing the world and our lives as we knew it; and I would soon learn to survive in life's *new normal*. Masks, social distancing, hand sanitizer, vaccines, and *zooming* were my just a few of my new survival tools.

Thankfully, God has been with me throughout my journey providing helper and heroes to bless me. First, of course, is my daughter and her husband who made life more bearable during this unique time by validating my decision to move near them. I also had two amazing real estate agents – one who sold my Wilmington town home in one week for top dollar, and the other agent who helped find my new home in Mebane, NC.

Despite getting all my ducks in a row and planning back up options to work around this pandemic predicament, there were a few hiccups along the way. My new Mebane house was not finished until April, but the buyers of my Wilmington house graciously agreed to let me rent from them until I was ready to move – how lucky I was!

One morning in late March, I leaned the moving company I had selected would not be able to accommodate me. Lesson learned -- expect the unexpected. Fortunately, another small company was waiting to assist me who did great work for the right price!

I soon learned I had awesome new neighbors in my new community. I found a new walking partner, and discovered their volunteer *Cat Rescue Squad* was heroic in getting my cat out of the storm drainage pipes. Plus, there are some really good cooks providing me with lots of home baked goodies.

Despite the many hardships and tragedies the pandemic threw at us, there were hidden silver linings to be discovered. I silently wept each night as the evening news announced the latest COVID-19 statistics of illnesses and deaths. I had family members, friends and neighbors affected by the virus and who had lost a family member to lung cancer. No one was spared. My nightly prayer list kept growing.

Yet, there were many blessings to be found. I kept up with my friendships through texting, emails, video chats, etc., as we experienced this new life. Luckily, I did not suffer from depression, anxiety or loneliness (thanks to my two cats) that was so prevalent during the year. I was able to arrange for my church's minister to marry my cousin's son and his fiancé in April, as they had to cancel their traditional June wedding.

My first great joy came from the engagement of my Chicago daughter, Julia, to her fiancé, Chris. Secretly, I had given him my mother's engagement diamond for him to reset and make into a new ring. This secret exchange happened during Christmas of 2019 –the last time I saw them in person. Chris used his cell phone to video his surprise proposal to Julia. Because I was unable to fly to Chicago to help Julia pick out a wedding dress, I suggested she let Chris's mom, Evelyn, be my stand in. She had three boys, so had never experienced the pleasure of bridal dress shopping. I sat comfortably in my house chair watching via video chat as Julia tried on dresses until we all agreed on the "one." It was a win- win for everyone and a September 2021 wedding was planned, in Chicago. Who knows – perhaps Julia's Springer spaniel, "Bonnie," will be the ring bearer!

My second great joy came in February of 2021 as I got both doses of the Pfizer vaccine and had no bad reaction to either shot. I was proud to tell everyone I was the first generation to get the polio vaccine in the 1950's, and now, I am in the first generation to get the Corona virus vaccine. I'm special! Fortunately, all of my family has now been vaccinated, but we still follow CDC safety guidelines.

The future is still a mysterious unknown to all of us. However, with faith and trust in God and the belief in power of positivity, we will continue surviving and finding the right answers to navigate this brave new world.

Michael Felder and His Dog in South Carolina, in his own Words

In fall of 2019 I had the good fortune to attend a service in the Episcopal Church in Jeffers. Jeffers is a small community with about 5 very nice houses that are well maintained. The cabin where we were staying was less than a mile from this church. It is a beautiful small church. There were about 15 people at the service and everyone knew each other. Near the end the "lay person" (the regular minister was away) who had given the sermon mentioned that there was a new person at the service. She asked if I might say who I was. I did say who I was and I was from Columbia, SC. A person sitting near me later said his college roommate was from Columbia and he had visited many times. After the service we had homemade cinnamon rolls and coffee. Everyone sat around tables and we just talked. This was a beautiful church inside and outside. The people were so genuine and seemed very happy. As I was leaving, one person left with me and wanted to show me

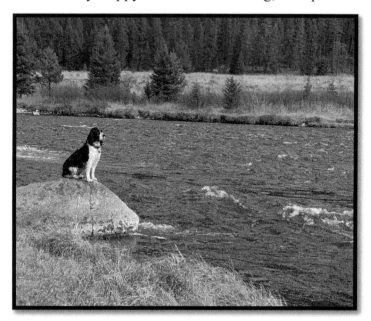

something. There was an embroidered Lord's Prayer behind a glass enclosure. It was approximately 2 feet by 3 feet. The person wanted me to see this as it had been done by his grandmother. I was looking forward to attending that church in 2020, but a blizzard and high winds came through and power was lost for about 12 hrs. There was no service the Sunday I was there. I was very disappointed that I could not see those people again.

Figure 64 K9 Emma.

164

My English Springer spaniel, Emma, and I have been traveling to Ennis, Montana to fish on the Madison River for a few years now. We went in early November 2020 and stayed for a week in a beautiful and rustic cabin with views of the mountains and an occasional deer or moose could be seen very near our cabin. I drive to Montana and it's a 32 hour trip. Emma is a very good dog to travel with and sleeps much of the time. I drive because I cannot think of risking her being transported by plane.

We had a good fishing experience catching quite a few nice brown and rainbow trout. Emma is very tough in the outdoors and does lots of running in the tall grass and I've seen her "springing" in the tall grass on occasion. I've never gotten a video of it but it's a beautiful thing to see.

Emma is a wonderful dog. She is spoiled, ha, but she is very tough and will jump in the Madison River and swim even with outside temp being below freezing. She tries to catch the trout when I'm trying to get them into a net. After that she paws in the water and thinks she can catch a fish. Emma is a fabulous dog. She is such a joy to have.

We have avoided any COVID-19 infection and were careful on the trip. Of course, fishing in a beautiful river with few other people is not a good place to contact the virus!!! We enjoy the drive although it is long. It's beautiful to see America and the farming areas of Illinois, Iowa, and South Dakota. America is a wonderful place and we are fortunate to live in a beautiful country. The farm houses always look so clean and well maintained. We enjoyed our trip and it was a wonderful way to experience the outdoors without much chance of catching the virus.

Michael Felder beautifully expressed in the article above, how life went on, nature was still enjoyed and animals helped us to maintain a sense of normalcy, often filling the void made by a lack of interaction with our fellow family and friends. As a matter of fact, English Springer spaniel breeders noted a huge demand for Springer puppies during the pandemic. It may be assumed this anomaly spread to other breeds as well, as families decided it was a good time to welcome a new puppy into the family. There is nothing like a family pet to distract and help us give the love inside to another living baby (human or not).

———

All of us were wondering what would come next. Will we get back to a normal routine and let the era of the COVID-19 slowly fade, albeit never leave, our memory. We were expecting acceleration in our state with community spread in North Carolina.

Before easing the restrictions, states were expected to have at least 14 days of declining numbers. So, we watched those statistics wondering if we will ever get back to normal.

We totally expected that social distancing at some level would become more of the norm. We wondered if we would ever get back to the packed stadiums, movie theaters, or large family gatherings. We suspected so but were not sure when that might happen.

We hoped for rapid testing when the individual and medical provider could get test results in less than an hour. We were looking for antibody testing so we could know for sure if we have had it or not and have antibodies to fight against it, if it reared its head again in our personal circle.

We hoped for a treatment such as antiviral therapy, serum therapy, and/or a combination of medications which could help the positive patient. We were weary of promises and fearful of side effects of a possible vaccine.

We continued to quarantine ourselves at home for 14 days if we traveled away from our home area. Here in Brunswick County, health advisors told us that we will not be tested if we are sick and feel we could continue at home. They told us we were still in the surge period and the highest of the curve may come in May.

At that time, April 7, 2020, we were still staying home. We were continuing with our hygiene routine, washing our hands so frequently that we were using up all the hand lotion. When we are out and about, visiting stores or such, we were constantly using the antibacterial hand spritzers to sanitize when returning to our cars. We were continuing social distancing and isolating ourselves if we were sick or had been around anyone sick.

We were still encouraged to call 911 if we had a shortness of breath, chest pain or pressure, blue lips, difficulty breathing or confusion. (Blue lips, seriously….difficulty breathing….well of course!!)

We continued to check on our friends and family calling them regularly to see how they were doing. If there was an unmet need, we were encouraged to call and let someone know at the county level so it might be provided. My friend, Jane Getty in New Jersey, visited a 96-year-old neighbor daily bringing her dogs on a six-foot lead to cheer her up. Jane never entered her home but from a distance allowed her to see her favorite dog, waved and chatted a bit.

We were encouraged to stay updated on the latest state and local guidelines and recommendations through media and web announcements. We continued to watch the nightly news to see if there is anything had changed. Mostly it had not.

The Three T's

The state governors and leaders were encouraged to make decisions based upon the Three T's. Here is the description of that plan as presented:

T: Testing

Testing for the presence of the virus and antibodies needs to be widely available with the focus on sending some of the testing to the general population.

On April 17th, 2020 Dr. Anthony Fauci stated on the nightly COVID-19 Task Force Briefing, *"There are two types of tests. One is to test if someone has been infected and recovered; and may be protected against future infections."*

"Then there is the test of whether or not you are infected which is a nucleic acid test and different types within that. It is a sensitive and specific test and if you are infected, you will know you are infected. If you get a test today, and it is negative, that does not mean that tomorrow or the next or the next day, and you get around someone who is positive, it does not mean you will stay negative."

"The other test is an antibody test and tells you if you have been infected and will give you a broader view, what the penetrance of the infection has been." "We need to know what is the titer of the protection…and we do not know if it is one month, one year, or longer." The difference between them is what we need it for us to identify, isolate and contact trace during Phase one."

"Testing is a part of a multifaceted way we will control this outbreak." "And if we do these things correctly, it will take this country safely through phase one."

Dr. Robert Redfield, CDC Director, at the same briefing, stated, "We are well-equipped to monitor the flu types and corona virus peaks and now in week 15 our flu surveillance system is really coming down." "There are more than 500 CDC officials throughout the states, and there will be additional personnel in states which request them."

Dr. Deborah Birx, COVID-19 Task Force Coordinator, explained that in regards to sampling for the virus itself, "the swabs put into your nose can diagnose and the antibody tests can show whether you have had the virus." "The asymptomatic monitoring of people who do not remember having any symptoms is now available." "Antibody tests have different specificity and sensitivity. The FDA has been very cautious about the antibody test and found they were 50 – 70% false. Those tests perform better when there is a high number of the virus around the states. They will be used around those high numbers areas to test the tests." In addition, Dr. Birx recommended that, "over 30 per 1000 population should be tested to get an idea of how many were or are affected."

Admiral Brett Giroir, HHS Assistant Secretary of Health, shared that, "Over 3 million tests have been administered in the U.S. as of April 16th. We have and will continue to have enough tests to enter Phase One of the re-entry plan."

"We will enter Phase One when there are 200,000 cases of the virus or less in the United States. This will require about 1 out of 10 people are tested, so we will need about 2 million tests. Each one who is positive has contacts which will need to be traced. The CDC says it is usually about 5 contacts. We need another million to trace the contacts. So now we need about 4 million tests done."

"The second group of testing fits with the surveillance system to monitor and test people who are asymptomatic. The strategy is to test about 300,000 to 500,000 people a week who are in the most vulnerable population such as nursing homes; and community health centers who take care of 30 million people, many below the poverty level. We also want to do our indigenous populations through the Indian Health Services. Totally, we will need to test a total of 4.5 million per month."

T: Tracing

Local health departments are setting up additional teams to trace anyone exposed and hope to rapidly do contract tracing so those individuals can be quarantined and isolated. They suspect more manpower will be needed to do this task and our state is looking for innovative ways to accomplish this.

T: Trends

Health Services will be looking at cases, hospitalizations and curves as we move through the highest surge and decline of cases.

Brunswick County is still having problems getting personal protective equipment such as gloves, masks and gowns, etc., from the state but are currently managing with what we have.

There is no word yet as to when North Carolina will ease the restrictions. There continues to be on-going planning.

Senate Help Committee Hearing. First Ever Senate Hearing with Witnesses & Chairman appearing remotely due to Pandemic Concerns held on May 12, 2020.

The first ever *Senate hearing* with witnesses and the chairman appearing remotely, due to the pandemic concerns, was held on **May 12, 2020**. The Chairman was Senator Lamar Alexander, from Tennessee who led the committee hearings. Participating and answering questions from the Senate Committee members were: *Dr. Anthony Fauci*, White House Task Force Committee, *Dr. Robert Redfield*, CDC (Center for Disease Control); *Stephen Hahn*, Commissioner of Food and Drug Administration, FDA (Federal Drug Administration); *Admiral Brett Giroir*, Asst. HHS Secretary (Heath and Human Services). Some of the questions and answers given during the hearing are included here for a general overview of the Senate concerns during this pandemic. Although a few comments and questions seemed quite political in nature, most were generally concerned about the pandemic and the state of affairs and are paraphrased in this section.

Vaccines are still in the process of being developed but not expected to be available to the general public for another 12 to 18 months. Senators interviewed Dr. Fauci on May 12th asking many questions about how this will proceed. He stated that even with the ones being developed there is no guarantee they will work. Several are being developed. The FDA and NIH are working together. During this interview, Senator Burr, of North Carolina, encouraged all to share the number of recovered persons in addition to the cases and death reports. He also encouraged all states to follow North Carolina in doing this.

Dr. Fauci had a basic concern about state and territory openings. "In an attempt to get back to normality, the checkpoints that we have put into our guidelines are there because re-opening too quickly provides a real risk that it will trigger another outbreak that you cannot control. Re-opening too early without guidelines could set us back on the road in order to get economic recovery. That is my major concern."

Questions about what was happening in nursing homes, especially where staff and patients had been affected so strongly and were particularly hard-hit were the theme of several senators. All nursing homes were required to report cases to the CDC.

Dr. Redfield answered questions about how employees and families are notified of cases within the nursing homes and long-term living facilities. He explained, "A national surveillance system is being implemented and CDC is doing that in conjunction with the states. Infection control procedures have been enhanced and CDC employees have been out across the nation to help with that."

Senator Rand Paul said, "Rhesus monkeys who are infected cannot be re-infected. Convalescent plasma can be beneficial as donated. Recovered COVID patients show significant antibody responses and produce an immunity for at least two to three years." According to Rand Paul, "the question of immunity is linked to health partners. The silver lining is that there are so many infections in the meat industry, that it is likely that they will not get it again. Please set the scientific record straight that if you have it, it will likely lead to immunity.

Dr Fauci said, "When you have antibody present, you very likely to have protection against re-infection. Long term historical studies or degree of protection are not yet available. In a period of months to years it will tell you definitely if that is the case; but in all likelihood, the vast majority will have immunity."

Rand said, "In reality evidence is stacking up and it is very unlikely you will get it again. Between the ages of 0 and 18, the mortality rate is 10 out of 100 thousand. What affects will this have on restarting school?" Rand went on to say, "We do no need to keep kids out of school for a year and I think it is a huge mistake if kids do not return to school in the fall."

Fauci responded, "We need to be very careful about what we do with children. We are seeing children presenting with COVID-19 that have a strange inflammatory respiratory affect. Children do much better than adults." Fauci said he is "very careful and humble that

169

he does not know everything about this disease and therefore careful about his predictions," when challenged about being the one who makes all the decisions about our nation's response to COVID-19. Fauci said he is a scientist and makes his "recommendations based on science and data, not personal opinion."

Senator Tammy Baldwin asked Dr. Redfield about the PPE (personal protective equipment) model being used at the White House. She asked, "In regards to the testing protocols present, is this model for other essential work places?" Dr. Redfield responded with, "Each workplace must define their own approach. CDC has put out guidelines of staying apart at least six feet and to wear face coverings." He refused to be baited into making a statement about many individuals from the White House not wearing face masks or coverings; at least when on television.

Admiral Brett Giroir, Asst. HHS Secretary, talked about "working with states and every lab in every state to increase capacity for testing. He said "Over the last few months, we have done a lot of work at meat packing plants, nursing homes, etc. Now we are working with the state leadership and state labs so that they can understand what the funding will be at their level." He went on to say, "In regards to delivery of supply: PPE, Testing, medical equipment, particularly for things like swabs for testing, there are too many variables to control; so, we are using manufacturers who are larger and represent more mature aspects of the industry, to make the swabs."

Senator Susan Collins asked Dr. Redfield, "I am hearing all over the state of Maine that the dentist cannot practice in our state, despite following infection protocols, and this is causing health problems for the dentists. Dental health is so important and Maine state officials are trying to make the right decisions. If dentists are following ADA (American Dental Association) guidelines, instituting protective measures for their patients and staff and self, and if closely examining data and seeing a decline in COVID-19 infections in their counties, are these reasonable factors to consider in reopening the practice of dentistry?" Dr. Redfield replied, "We have been working with state and local officials to update our guidelines for a variety of medical services. I would not disagree with what you said about looking at the ADA associations and the coming updates will include dental guidelines."

Senator Collins asked Dr. Giroir and Dr. Hahn questions in regards to the medication *remdesivir* and the authorization to use it. She said, "Maine hospitals, specifically two of the largest hospitals, have questions about how these will be allocated going forward. Will these emergency allocations go to states instead of hospitals...distribution plans are not clear. Each state is expected to receive some allocation but no timetable is provided. I am concerned that hospitalized patients in Maine will have no ability to be treated in the foreseeable future. Can these and ultimately vaccine allocations and distribution issues be resolved so that patient care is not delayed?"

Dr. Hahn replied, "We must be an evidence-based approach to get the medications to the patients in need. This is led by HHS (Health and Human Services). The Task Force provided guidance where the most significant outbreaks and hospitalized patients were located."   Adm. Giroir said, "I have nothing to add.   I agree with Commissioner Hahn…evidence based on the people who can benefit from it."

Senator Patty Murray from Washington, asked if the three doctors who are in quarantine, Dr Fauci, Dr. Redfield, and Dr. Hahn, are all drawing a salary during your period of quarantine. Dr. Fauci responded, "We are essential workers and when needed are available. It is not strictly quarantine, but performing our duties as critical workers."

"Dr Stephen Hahn said, "Yes, we are drawing our salary and will continue to meet face-to-face when critical." Murray continued with, "My point is that quarantine is easy for people like you and me, but there are millions of Americans who work jobs that cannot be paid for by working at home or work by the hour; and we need a quarantine system for all Americans; but my state has no clue how to pay for this."

"There are dangers of states opening too early. The President has said we prevailed over coronavirus but you are saying (Fauci) that we may be opening too early. I worry that you are trying to have it both ways. But then you don't give us the resources to succeed. The President may be undermining your guidance. The plan to reopen America was meant to be followed with a downward trajectory. What happens if you re-open and have a spike? And have you developed specific guidance that will be helpful? We don't have all the experts you have. Was this guidance that was developed by you and other experts shelved by decisions made in the White House? Why didn't this plan get released and when or if it will be? We need this additional guidance," said Senator Murray.

Dr. Redfield responded, "We have developed a series of guidance as you know. As we work through the guidance plans, they go through interagency review to be more broadly applicable to society, and come back to CDC; and back to the Task Force for review. CDC stands by the technical assistance to your state and any state, at their request, and has posted information on the CDC website. Your state can reach out to CDC and we will give guidance on any issue."

Senator Bill Cassidy of Louisiana asked Dr. Hahn, "All trials include the most vulnerable, younger, etc. Are you assessing the safety in children?" He wanted to know if the FDA and NIH are discussing whether this will include children. He was concerned with school openings and modifications which may be needed. Will we have targeted testing? There are no guidelines about how to integrate testing in schools." Dr. Redfield said, "Clearly there will be a testing strategy in different school settings and locations; general guidelines and testing strategy and surveillance strategy needs to be individualized. Elementary, high school, college trade school may have different options for guidance. These will be coming."

Senator Cassidy asked Dr. Fauci: "I have concerns about missing school, brain development, and the unintended consequences of having to do something different as a result of the virus. Dr. Fauci said, "There is no easy answer and we have to see, on a step by step basis in the fall, where we are at that time. We have a large country and dynamics are different in one region versus another and answers will not be homogeneous. We have no answers to when we close schools and it presents based on various circumstances."

Senator Elizabeth Warren, from Massachusetts stated, "Over 1.3 million are infected; about 80,000 have died, and 33 million are out of work. Dr. Fauci, you have advised six presidents. What is your honest opinion, do we have the corona virus contained?" Dr. Fauci answered with, "Under control, we do not. We have an increase of hospitalizations in some parts of country and some are coming down. The trend looks flat with some coming down. We are going in the right direction but it does not mean we have total control of this infection." Warren said that "some estimated we could be at 200,000 new cases by June." Dr. Fauci responded with, "I do not believe that and we will be much better than that."

Senator Maxine Waters, of California said, "We are 3 months into this pandemic and we are setting records of the number of people who get it and die. We are 16 weeks away from Labor Day. Do we have enough counter measures in place so we do not have to worry about a bad fall? Dr Fauci said, "Projection is that by the time we get to early fall, we will have testing and contact tracing in place. If we do an adequate response, we will be ok. If we do not respond in an adequate way, in the fall, we run the risk of resurgence. But I hope that by that time we will have enough testing and contact tracing." Warren: The virus is not yet under control. President needs to stop pretending that if he ignores bad news it will go away. He needs to respond. We are running out of time to save lives. Urgency of the moment is not being met."

Senator Pat Roberts of Kansas stated, "We must be bipartisan or we will not get anywhere. We are the hot spot in Kansas because of a few meatpacking plants. We have a large cattle market. We should be worried about the food supply which is in great distress. Agriculture has stepped up. Packing plants are a national asset here in Dodge City. Problems in agriculture and our relationship with China, seems to be on hold. I am worried that the food value chain is very real and a financial situation that farms and ranchers are facing. There are five packing plants in Kansas…can we get a rapid test? For this hot spot?"

Admiral Giroir said, "Dr. Redfield and I are involved in getting strategies for the industry, particularly in Kansas by supplying public health labs with rapid diagnostics. In regards to the rapid point of care diagnostics…each machine can only do 4 per hour and that is very slow. Quest lab in Kansas can help with a solution and CDC is on the ground in Kansas." Senator Roberts said, "As we reopen, we have contingency plans that if the re-opening plans don't work, and it will be a tough go, and in terms of agriculture, we are not in good shape."

Senator Tim Kaine from Virginia compared the statistics of the United States and South Korea on three specific dates noting that the economy of South Korea has not changed at all. He compared the death rates and per capita said that the U.S. has 45 times the death toll as South Korea. He continued with more statistics from other countries. "So, to Dr. Fauci, the death toll in the U.S., especially when compared to other nations is unacceptable, isn't it?" Dr. Fauci, "Yes, of course, the death rate that high in any manner of form is unacceptable. We always have to do better." Kaine stressed that there is a big difference between South Korea and America and the outbreak. South Korea began aggressive testing much earlier than we did during the critical month of March. South Korea was testing at a rate of 40 X the U.S. He said, "We need to learn from those who did it right."

Senator Lisa Murkowski of Alaska discussed assistance to Alaska and thanked the committee members for all they have done. "So much of focus has been on hotspots, but we need to help small rural communities. Are we doing enough? Travel restrictions are working but devastating our economy." Admiral Giroir said, "You have a good protocol of keeping Alaska safe. We are working with your state to meet challenging testing requirements as you cannot send out labs a thousand miles away. There is a comprehensive strategy in Alaska. Given circumstances, we understand the challenge in the fishing and remote environment but all have to come together to keep your environment safe. Many of your community were almost annihilated in the 1918 pandemic and we need to give them all the protection we can."

Senator Murkowski said, "Contact tracing is the key in getting back to school and work. We have teams in place. What more do we need to be doing, once you are tested positive on contact tracing? I am not convinced we are focusing enough on this." "Contact tracing is critical and is the difference between succeeding and containing the virus from wide scale spread and we are positioning to deploy about 500 CDC officials; but most importantly, we are trying to work with your health department; with the census bureau and labs, to develop your testing and contact tracing. This will take a significant effort and augmented. We are there to work with the states," Redford replied.

Senator Maggie Hassan, from New Jersey said that we need leadership from the CDC and public health experts.

Senator Tim Scott, of South Carolina noted "For those older Americans and those with chronic conditions, this virus remains a threat; a dangerous threat. In SC the medium age of those who died was 76.5; nearly 2/3s were older than 71, and 90% were over the age of 60; 98% were over the age of 50. Every death is a tragedy. We are taking every measure to protect our older South Carolinians and those with underlying conditions. We knew it was impossible to set out to avoid 100% fatalities. At same time mental and physical health declines. Businesses collapsed. We are waiting for good news and flattening the curve. We need to do better and will do better. As we move toward reopening, what else can we do to protect our most vulnerable populations?"

Dr. Fauci replied, "You have put things in place to optimize your capability of reopening. Vulnerable populations, as we have said in our guidelines, are ready to progress carefully. The vulnerable should be the very last to lift mitigations. In other words, protect them up until the very end as those individuals are the most vulnerable. Those in the minority groups, Hispanics and blacks have a greater capacity of getting infected but have a higher risk because of underlying factors." Scott said, "Without any questions, typically African Americans and Hispanics are providing care in the nursing homes."

Senator Tina Smith, of Minnesota, asked Dr. Fauci, "How are you holding up?" He said, "I am really fine. Thank you for asking. It transcends all of us individually and working as a team. I am fine and I appreciate your concern. We are grateful for your service and all of you." Smith went on to say, "Agriculture, pork processors, are looking at reality of euthanizing thousands of hogs a day because there are no places to process them because of the workers getting sick in the processing plants. As we think about how we move forward, what guidance do you give us?"

Dr. Fauci said, "Not the area of my expertise. It would seem like if you want to keep packing plants open, you have to provide the optimum protection for workers involved and go to work safely; and, if infected, get them out immediately, and get them immediate care. There is the responsibility to take care of them. This is not an official proclamation but my recommendations as a doctor and human being. Senator Smith said, "This is the kind of guidance we should be getting and following and the tools we need in our country if we want to open our economy." Dr. Fauci continued, " One of things I emphasize is that when you are in the process of pulling back mitigation and opening up, you must have the capability to respond when you have a uptake in infections to rebound or it will set us back in our progress of opening up the country."

Senator Mitt Romney, Utah, questioned the testing processes of South Korea and the United States saying, "Our testing record is nothing to celebrate. There are lessons for us as we think about for the future. With regards to vaccines, we have done a pretty darn good job moving ahead aggressively. Is President Obama or Trump responsible that we do not have a vaccine now or delaying it in some way?"

Fauci replied, "No, neither is responsible for not having a vaccine. We are moving rather rapidly in going from knowing there is a virus to what we have done." Romney continued, "Accurate data is not there on a day-to-day basis, in the CDC." Dr. Redfield explained that day-to-day analysis needs to be improved. Funding for data modernization is forthcoming and we are in the process of implementing that. "One problem is non-integrated public health systems in place. This country needs predictive analysis and is one of the shortcomings we have identified and we need time to get that corrected."

Senator Romney asked, "Dr. Fauci, one last thing…we are all hoping for a vaccine and the objective of our administration as soon as we can; given our history how likely is it we will get a vaccine within a year or two or is it a long shot?" Fauci said, "Definitely not a long shot and more likely we will. Overwhelmingly people recover although there is morbidity among certain populations. From a conceptual standpoint, we can stimulate the body to produce a similar response…somewhere within that time frame."

Senator Doug Jones, of Alabama had a question for Dr. Redfield, "Contract tracing, I understand you are working with states to develop plans for re-opening. Using that data will be important in terms of child care facilities, facilities like hotels and motels, to use for self-isolation. Are the plans individualized by state? In congress, will we have access to these plans? How will these plans be developed and what access will we have to see these plans?"

Dr. Redfield said, "It is a critical component to develop contact tracing prior to fall. Discussions have already happened about contact tracing. We have over 500, possibly additional personnel being brought in to help states, to help them hire contact tracing help. AmeriCorps and Peace Corps will also help to develop the contact tracing piece. We have also used military bases to use as isolation procedures. There is a certain capacity that is intrinsic like motels, individuals who need to self-isolate when in a multi-family home or large families. We need to identify cases and then do the appropriate public health measure. I see no reason why they cannot be transparent documents. 1.6 billion dollars have been put into the states for this. It is important, highly functional plan to contain the virus and not have to switch into mitigation."

Senator Mike Braun of Indiana posed a question to Dr. Hahn. "When we first met, will the FDA be able to help the healthcare system in general? Has the administration ever put an impediment in developing testing during the January 24 to March 5th time span? Early testing was created and the CDC was going to do their own tests; and South Korea test would not be used. Long and short of all of this, nearly a month, this was in a bureaucratic swirl. CDC denied access to functioning tests in South Korea."

Dr. Hahn responded, "We will look at every one of our regulatory authorities and provided significant flexibility to allow developers to ensure the gold standard of safety and will continue to learn and commit the changes that are necessarily and still protect the safety of all medical products.

Senator Braun asked Dr. Fauci, "Can we do it for COVID-19 like you put into place with HIV/Aids, the protocol you put into place then in the 90s?" Fauci responded with, "It is a different story with some similarities. In the late 80s, there was no availability for HIV and we were testing drugs; and in that protocol we would make it available for compassionate use because there was a dire need for accessibility for those drugs. For some who needed a chance, it was outside of the protocols. Compassionate use. This is a version that has not yet been fully proven; drugs, and what we did then and what we are doing now." Dr. Hahn added, "Emergency Use authorization process allows flexibility in a public health emergency and we continue to look at those requests when they come in."

Senator Jacky Rosen from Nevada, said "Casinos, restaurants, and attractions must feel confident our visitors are safe; and we need a vaccine and understand this takes time. What research is happening regarding preventable treatments before the vaccine is available? What is happening to identify potential antibody preventative medication to block COVID19 from latching on? Are preventive medications effectiveness or vaccines available?"

Fauci said, "In all medications being developed, that is just one of the possibilities being developed; plasma, preventive modalities are feasible, and will be pursued which are parallel with the development of the vaccine. Many interventions of preventing HIV/Aids were worked in parallel and will be a part of the effort at the same time as we are trying to get a vaccine."

Senator Rosen asked, "What does our next generation need to look like for all of us as we go about our life? Airplane, out to eat, etc.? PPE for the general public?" Dr. Fauci maintained that the "best PPE is maintaining physical and social distancing. All agree that it is beyond your control when you need to do necessary things…grocery store, drug store. This is the reason why some time ago, the CDC, recommended some sort of covering or facial mask. For the time being, PPE should be a regular part of preventing spread of infection. Many people are wearing masks and this gives me a degree of comfort that people are taking this seriously."

Senator Kelly Loeffler, of Georgia focused her questions with, WHO, global health questions, and needed reforms. Loeffler was concerned about a cover up of information from China in their efforts to suppress information at the outbreak. She feels we need to take steps to ensure that another outbreak cannot take hold in this way. She asked Dr. Redfield about his level and timing of information from his Chinese counterparts as this virus emerged. Dr. Redfield explained, "The CDC has had relationships from countries around world, 45 countries, one is China. We at the CDC, with the Chinese CDC, have worked together for decades, collaboratively. When this original outbreak came from wet markets, I had discussions on January 3, to discuss this on the scientific level. We had good interactions. That is different from the broader government level."

Senator Loeffler said, "The mainstream media wants to paint your relationship as controversial with our president. Can you address this? What is the characterization and true or untrue? Fauci answered, "There is certainly not a controversial relationship between me and the President. I give advice based on scientific information and he gets information from others. Never has there been a confrontational situation between us." Redfield added, "We are there to give our best public health device grounded in data and science. It is done in professional way and I echo Dr. Fauci. I have not had a confrontational relationship with the president and he has listened." "Admiral Giroir said, "I echo my colleagues. We work very closely and have a productive relationship with each other and the President and Vice President. We have the ability to honestly state our opinions and recommendations and it has been that way from the beginning."

Senator Patty Murray of Washington, was concerned with it being crucial that clinical trials recognize racial and ethnic disparities which have been overlooked and unacknowledged. Dr. Fauci said, "Racial and ethnic concerns in clinical trials will be representatives in minority and populations at most risk." It is something we started back in the days of HIV and we will do that with these trials." Dr. Hahn added, "The FDA vaccine developers and the NIH efforts work together and have data transparency between the manufacturers and NIH, so we can understand the capacity and supply chain. Five to seven vaccines are being developed." Senator Murray said, "There is more work to do before we can get back to work and school and some semblance of normalcy. We need the White House to lay out a plan. We still need PPE when the time comes. We still need guidance from our experts so our states have the knowledge to open up and keep our community safe. We have a lot more to do. Thank you to all for joining us today."

The chairman of the committee, Senator Lamar Alexander, clarified: "Dr. Fauci said vaccines are coming as fast as they ever have but it will be later in the year. There are some treatments that are modest but could be more. That does not mean you should not go back to school." Dr. Fauci added that, "Going back to school would be more in the realm of knowing the landscape and depend upon the dynamics of the outbreak where the school is. There is no relationship in the available of a vaccine and going back to school."

Senator Alexander said, "Ramping up tests availability should be adequate for school officials to test every student in the school if they need to. 40 to 50 million tests will be available a month, in about three months; and will be available depending upon the dynamics of the area. Keep sanitation, personal cleanliness; face masks, etc. in place. For 100,000 schools and 5,000 campuses, testing and commonsense hygiene can be used to plan for school opening in August. In the National Plan, "There is a push and tug as to what is national and federal and what states should do. The law actually requires states to tell federal what their plans are. What Washington does and what states do is sometimes in debate. Strategy is led by governors and designed by a national effort. National efforts are of a vaccine development." "We reiterate that this hearing has been helpful. We are impressed by the diversity of opinion from senators and four remarkable participants." "As we deal with this pandemic, we need to be sure we are ready for the next one and stockpile for the next one."

Chairman, Lamar Alexander, from Tennessee, of the Senate Help Committee concluded, "We need to deal with this crisis and also deal with the next one, THIS YEAR. Our job is to create an environment where states succeed and this creates a country that succeeds." The three-hour hearing was concluded with lots of snippets for the media to discuss. And another day was done.

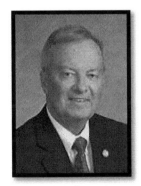

Representative Frank Iler[75], of the North House of Representatives said, "A state committee is looking at pushing back some due dates such as tax due dates to July 15th when they get back into session. The committee is also looking into how to help our citizens with some of the state 'rainy-day' funds and what purchases need to be made for future preparedness."

Figure 65 Rep. Frank Iler.

The House of Representatives will be back in session the week of April 28th, 2020, where all of these will come into discussion.

---

[75] Frank Iler is a Republican member of the North Carolina House of Representatives representing the state's seventeenth House district, covering portions of Brunswick County, North Carolina. A retired businessman who lives on Oak Island, North Carolina, Iler was appointed when Bonner L. Stiller resigned in 2009.

Dealing with the Virus and Losing a Loved One

Amid all of the confusion and anxiety, everyone dealt with the virus in their own way. Many lost their loved ones to the COVID-19 virus. Connie Ivey was just one of over 500 million who has a story of Covid destroying lives. Mrs. Ivey's story is shared by her husband, Gerald Ivey, of Holden Beach, North Carolina.

My Story - By Gerald Ivey of Holden Beach, NC

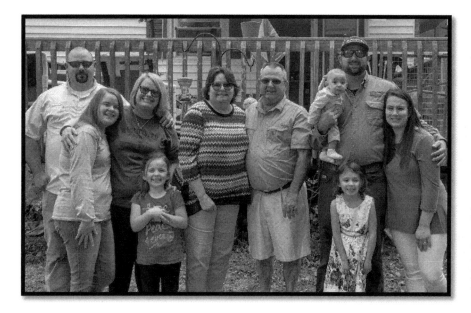

Figure 66 The Ivey Family.

Center: Connie & Gerald Ivey. Sons, Will and Gerik Ivey and their families.

On July 29th, 2020, I lost my wife of forty years to the COVID-19 virus. Her name was Connie Ivey. We lived at Holden Beach North Carolina.

That year was supposed to be a year of celebrations. The pandemic changed that. We had already started planning how we were going to celebrate our fortieth wedding anniversary on April 27th. The one thing that Connie enjoyed was getting together with family and friends.

Connie and I grew up together. We met at a little church name Union Chapel at a youth meeting. She was 12 and I had just turned 14; we were so young. We dated though high school and after I finished college while Connie was still in the 12th grade, we got married. Our love for each other grew as the years went by.

Being able to celebrate our fortieth anniversary was a big deal. The disappointment of not being able to have a big gathering didn't outweigh the risk of getting the virus. With the death toll climbing, we decided that because of the health risks that Connie and I already had, that it was best to keep our distance. Our two sons, Will and Gerik, would bring the grandkids to the front yard so Connie and I could see them.

May 12th was another mile stone for us. I turned 60 years old, and again the disappointment of not being able to celebrate with family and friends didn't outweigh the risk. Connie because of her health issues for several years was battling severe depression and the isolation wasn't helping.

The reports regarding the virus were only getting worst. Businesses were being forced to shut down. Schools were closed. Because of my employment, I was deemed essential and we were allowed to stay open. I would make sure to wash my hands and change clothes when I got home trying to make sure that I didn't bring the virus to Connie.

We would use separate bathrooms to try to keep the risk down. Connie had cancelled her doctor appointments and the ones that couldn't be cancelled were done by Zoom. My family did what was right to make sure that Connie and I were kept safe from the virus.

Unfortunately on Friday, June 19th I came home from work with a severe headache and by Saturday I started a mild fever and lost my taste and sense of smell. I quarantine myself away from Connie praying that she would not start having any symptoms. On Sunday June 21st Connie started running a fever. Our fears had come to realization. With all the horrible news that was being reported, Connie and I knew what this meant. We held on to each other and prayed. Monday June 22nd we both got tested and quarantine ourselves from everyone. We got a call on the 25th that Connie and I had tested positive for COVID-19. I called my work to inform them only to find out that there were more employees that had the virus also.

I called the doctor because Connie was getting confused and my O2 level was starting to drop. On June 26th the doctor called and wanted Connie and I to go to the hospital to be admitted. I told Connie that I didn't want to be in the hospital; that if I was I couldn't keep up with her. Against what she wanted I took her to the emergency room.
When we got there we had to wait for the nurse to come get Connie. We held on to each other and cried not knowing if we would ever see each other again.

That was the hardest thing I have ever had to do: leaving Connie by herself, after forty-four years. I have always been there for her and now because of the hospital policies, I couldn't. I returned back home because I was still under quarantine and not doing well myself.

My doctor called and wanted me to reconsider the decision that I made to not be admitted to the hospital. I told him that I feared that I could not keep up with Connie. I knew that I needed to try to be strong for her.

We were able to talk on the phone for a couple of days. She was so concerned about me; she wanted me to go to the ER. The last time I was able to talk to her was on June 29th. She was so confused.

I would call the hospital to get updates and the policies that the hospital had in place made it very hard to find out anything. The nurse was giving the task of giving the updates to the families. I felt like every time that I called that I was taking the nurse away from their patient's one being my wife, Connie.

The pain of not knowing how my wife of forty years was doing outweighed the guilt of calling the nurses. I wished the hospital had not put the task of speaking to the families on the nurses. They were on the front lines fighting for their patients and at the same time trying to be safe from this unknown killer.

June 30th I started reaching out by social media for prayers for Connie and I. My oxygen levels had dropped very low. My doctor would call everyday checking on me. He still wanted me to be admitted to the hospital but I knew I couldn't. I had to keep up with Connie.

July 1st my fever broke and oxygen levels started climbing, Praise the Lord. I kept reaching out by Facebook for people to pray and intercede for Connie.

July 2nd I received a phone call from the county that I was off quarantine. On July 3rd Connie's condition worsened. She was now on a ventilator and placed in the Intensive Care Unit. The pain of not being able to see her was so overwhelming and unbearable. I could only trust God.

I kept reaching out to the community giving updates so they could pray specifically for Connie's needs as they were getting worst. July 3rd, Friday afternoon, I received a call from the hospital that they were transferring Connie from Novant in Supply to New Hanover Hospital in Wilmington. I asked the hospital that since I was no longer in quarantine or contagious could I see my wife. I was told *no* and the hospital policies would not allow it.

I called and asked my sons, Will and Gerik, to take me to the hospital. We arrived and waited where the transport vehicle would be picking up Connie. When they pulled in, I asked them if I could see my wife. I was given permission (not that they were going to stop me). They said yes and I was able to see Connie when they came out with her. I kissed her on the forehead and told her that I loved her. She didn't respond but I know that she knew because we have showed each that we love each other every day for forty four years. I was glad that I got that moment with her.

I would give the updates everyday; most of the time twice a day. It was amazing the support and strength that my family and I were receiving though the prayers from my Pastor and church family and the many prayer warriors throughout this small community. They all had united together in Prayer and God was answering.

I was doing much better, still weak and short on breath, but was very thankful that I had survived the virus. Sunday, July 5th, the first update was positive. For the first time Connie was making small steps forward. I was so thankful and just like that my phone rang. It was Connie's doctor. He told me that Connie had suffered a major stroke and she needed surgery immediately. He continued to tell me that Connie will not survive without the surgery and there were a high probability that she would not survive the surgery. Again, I asked could I go see her, and, again I was denied. The emotional rollercoaster was so difficult and the pain was so real.

Connie survived the surgery. They were able to put a stint in and get blood flowing back to her brain. Connie had sustained major brain damage; to what extent the doctors didn't know yet.

Monday, July 6th, Connie was taken to have another CT scan. It was determined that the stroke was still evolving. They said Connie was not in any pain but that she seemed comfortable. Connie was in God's hands, my prayer for Connie changed that day. I started praying that God's wishes would be granted.

The waiting, the not knowing, was so difficult. All I could do was ask God for strength, peace and comfort. There are times in our lives when we can't pray because the hurt is so overwhelming. This was one of those times. I thank my Lord and Savior for showing up. He knows our needs even when we can't tell Him. I thank all the *Prayer Warriors* that were interceding on our behalf.

I returned back to work to try to keep my mind straight. I was thinking that if something happened I would already be near the hospital. Even though I was at work, my mind and heart was on Connie.

Tuesday, July 7th, it has been 12 days since Connie was admitted in the hospital. It seemed like months. I called the nurse for an update. She said they are taking small steps bringing the ventilator down. Connie was still requiring a high oxygen flow. The nurse asked if I wanted to see her. Praise the Lord, my prayers were going to be answered but not in the way I thought.

The nurse set up a Zoom call for Tuesday afternoon. The anticipation of finally getting to see my wife was getting to me. Will she know me after the stroke? The time came and I called in. We couldn't get the sound to work, but let me tell you what happened. When Connie saw me on the laptop both of her big brown eyes opened wide and she started picking her hand up and waving it to me. Praise the Lord. Connie knew me.

The doctors didn't know what kind of response I would get or if I would get a response at all. But Connie recognized me. I was so happy and thankful.

Over the next few days the doctors tried to take Connie off the ventilator but were unsuccessful. July 11th, Saturday, Day 16, Connie passed the breathing test and her fever dropped some. Connie, for the first time since the stroke, initiated communication herself. Connie waved her hand indicating that she was hot. Hopefully, things were changing, finally toward the good.

By Saturday afternoon Connie was removed from the ventilator. Now the doctors can start checking the effect that the stroke had. July 14th, Connie was still in critical condition. The stroke has caused major brain damage. Most of her right side of the brain was not functioning. She was paralyzed on her left side and not able to speak or swallow.

I knew that God could still heal Connie.   I kept reaching out to the community for prayer support.   I also knew and prayed that Connie's wishes would be granted. July 17th the nurse set up another Zoom call. I was hoping for the same response that I got the first time. That didn't happen. Connie was struggling now, not being able to swallow or cough and it had caused pneumonia to set in.

I was still trying to work but now my breathing was getting difficult. I went to the doctor and they did x-rays, I was told that I needed to be admitted in the hospital that I had double pneumonia. What was I supposed to do? My wife was dying and I was hoping to get to see her again. I once again told my doctor I couldn't and that I had to try to see Connie one more time. July 23rd, the 28th day, the doctor called and told me that Connie condition was failing fast and she probably had only a couple of days left. I asked if I could see her, and again I was denied. I very angry and told the doctor that I was on my way to see my wife. I called Will to take me to the hospital. He asked me if they were finally going to let me see Connie. I told him that the doctor said his mama was dying and I wanted to try to get to see her.

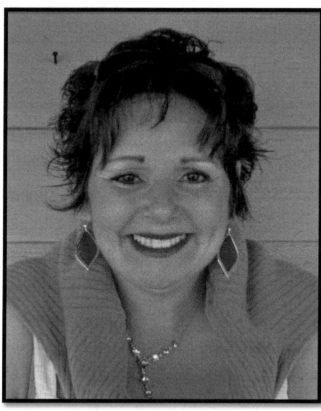

Figure 67 Connie Ivey.

Before Will could get home from his work, the doctor called twice. First he said that I could see her for 10 minutes and then called back the second time in ten minutes and said that Connie was no longer contagious and if I wanted to I could bring her home. *Thank you, Jesus.* I was going to see Connie again.

When I agreed the doctor prepare me for what to expect when I see Connie. The doctor said that Connie has not responded in the last two days and she was having regular seizures. The doctor asked me again if I still wanted to bring Connie home. There was only one answer. I called my family and they jumped in and got things ready.

I told Will and Gerik about Connie's condition to prepare them. When they got Connie home and brought her in the front door, I called out to her and told her that she was

182

home. Connie immediately opened both eyes and reached her right hand up to mine. The transport team was amazed. They said she has not responded at all. Thank you, Lord, for giving Connie strength to know that her family was there for her. He allowed us to talk with her.

Connie was a singer and had made a CD with her favorite songs. At the beginning of the CD Connie made a comment saying that these are the songs that has gotten her though many hardships. After we got Connie settled in the bed, I played her CD. Connie turned her head as much as she could and lifted her hand toward the Lord. I knew that Connie was drawing strength and comfort listening to her own voice singing to the Lord. I played it nonstop for the remaining of Connie's life.

Connie was able to respond for a couple of days squeezing my hand and moving her eyes. On July 29th at 7:09 in the morning, Connie received her total healing. She was made whole. Connie's suffering was over. She was now rejoicing with her love ones that had gone on before her. We had Connie's funeral on Friday, July 31st. She was buried at Union Chapel the same little church where I met that little brown-eyed girl forty-six years earlier. We got saved there before we were married in 1980.

On the headstone that was installed on Nov.3rd, Connie's birthday, you will see a picture of the last time that Connie and I held hands before she reach up and took Jesus' hand.

I miss her every day. I know that I will see her again. It's hard to believe that it has been over seven months since Connie went to her Heavenly home. It seems like yesterday. My life changed that day. I am still searching for my new identity. It has always been Connie and Gerald.

The following are the actual updates that I wrote on social media. You will see and feel my heart and pain. What you don't see are all the responses from my family, my pastor and this small community as they stood united in prayer. That got me and my family though the most difficult time in our life. Prayer moves the hand of God. When the doctor said that Connie was not responsive and only had a couple of days to live, God put strength back into her life and she knew that she was loved and at home. With all the uncertainties that 2020 brought upon all of us, one thing is for certain: God is still God.

There are three vaccines out now, and with the speed at which they were developed, there are a lot of people reluctant to take the shot. I get that, but I also know that if I could have avoided bringing the virus to my beautiful and loving wife I would have been in the front of the line. I would never wish this hurt on anyone. If you get anything from my story know this: God cares for you and we are blessed to live in a community that cares.

I will be fine. I am still battling with lung issues caused from the virus. Hopefully and prayerfully that will soon be healed but the broken heart will never be the same. I will always trust my Lord. I will draw strength from my Lord and Savior. I will wrap myself around my family and I will never let my grandchildren forget about their Nana. May God Bless *you*.

(Authors note: The following internet posts are printed just as they appeared online in their entirety.)

**These are the updates on Connie that I (Gerald Ivey) posted on the computer, via the program Facebook, during the hardest days that he had ever faced.

June 30th: We need to speak this prayer over Connie Ivey. We Declare and Speak life and command those lungs to BREATHE with the Breath of Life in Jesus Name. We release our Faith Now for Connie to rise up and be healed in Jesus Name!!!! Now...

We command this affliction from the enemy to go NOW in Jesus Name!!!! Connie hear the Word of God and rise up to life!!!!! In Jesus Name!!

Thanks Leonor Rueda Powell, This is what I have been hearing all day from different prayer warriors. Everyone needs to speak life over Connie, no matter what it looks like: Speak Life.

July 1[t]: Thanks for all the prayers that are being spoken for Connie, She has not had a good day, her oxygen levels continue to fall. I have to trust my Lord and Savior and stand upon His Word.

She is very weak and struggling for every breath, I promised her that I would never leave her and that I would be there always and because of the virus I am not able to fulfill that promise to her. I love her with all my heart. Connie I am so sorry that I brought this evil virus home to you; you are the love of my life. Please come back to me. This is so hard.

July 2nd: Update on Connie, First thanks for all your prayers, please continue to speak only positive words over Her, Her oxygen levels have continued to drop, she is now on 90 pct, if they lower it her levels drops to nearly nothing. She is however still responsive and eating. Prayers are sustaining her. As everyone knows or can imagine being away from her and not able to hold her though this is very hard, BUT let me tell you what the Comforter (Holy Spirit) has been doing. The nurse shared with me that every time she when in to check on Connie, she was having a conversation. The nurse said the first couple of times she didn't ask who Connie was talking to. After hearing this several times the nurse asked Connie. Who are you talking to? Connie's response was I am talking to my husband, he is right there. I have been so worried about Connie being scared and alone. And the Comforter has been there the whole time. That is the peace that no man can explain. I sit here at my home knowing that my wife is in His hands. Thanks and I look forward to the day that Connie is back with her family.

July 3rd: Update on Connie, she has taken a turn for the worst, they had to move her to the ICU and place her on a ventilator, Pray that while she is on the ventilator her heart will strengthen and the meds can begin to turn this horrible virus away. The county has finally released me from being isolated. I know I can't be with Connie but as I said in the previous post The Holy Spirit is her Comforter. Thanks for ALL the prayers.

July 4th: Update on Connie, she was transferred to New Hanover yesterday she is in the ICU in critical condition, she is still on the ventilator, right now she is stable. Thanks for all your prayers and support. It's during times like this that makes us stronger. Continue to speak the Word over Connie. There is power in the Word of God. The Holy Spirit is her Comforter and Jesus Christ is her Healer. I wish everyone a Happy 4th of July. Enjoy your family and always remember the reason we can.

July 5th am: Update on Connie She is making steps in the right direction. Thanks for all your prayers and support, PTL.

July 5th pm: This morning Connie had a massive stroke and a blood clot in her brain and was sent to emergency surgery. She came through surgery and is in recovery. They were able to put a stent in and get blood flow back to her brain. She does have brain damage but are not sure to what extent. Please continue to pray.

July 6th am: Update on Connie, the stroke is still evolving CT scan shows that the damage is worsening as the day goes. She is not in any pain and they are keeping her comfortable. Connie is in God's hands. My prayer for her is that The Lord will grant Connie her wishes. Pray that I will be able to see here again. I love you Connie Ivey

July 6th pm: Cannot get an update on Connie, Said they will try to call by 10, I wish the hospitals would put more thought in their process. Nurses should not be responsible for having to give families updates. They are the ones on the battlefield. The hospital should have someone designated to give the families updates.

July7th am: Update on Connie as of 6 am this morning... she is stable, they were able to bring the ventilator down some. They have not done another CT yet since yesterday, probably will do one this morning to see if the stroke is still evolving.

Thanks for all your prayers and support. We serve a Big God of mercy and grace. He knows our hearts. He knows our needs, and Our Lord and Savior Jesus Christ CARES. God bless each one of you and please remember my bother in Christ, Ray Patty Leazer, in your prayers also. He needs God's touch.

July 7th pm: Update on Connie... The nurse connected us up to the Zoom. We couldn't get the sound but I did get to see the Love of my life and let tell you what happened. When Connie opened an eye and saw that it was me on the other side, both of those big brown eyes of hers opened as big as quarters and she started opening and closing her right hand very fast. Not only did she recognize me but she was waving her hand. Thank you, Lord, for allowing this moment in time. My Heart is so overwhelmed, my soul is rejoicing. Praise the Lord for this golden nugget.

July 8th am: Update on Connie... After being able to Zoom with Connie at around 10 Tuesday morning and God blessing me with that golden nugget, I just received an update at 1 am this morning. Connie is stable and with no changes. They have made some baby steps with the ventilator. She is still able to follow commands on her right side only. But one thing I know, Connie recognized me on that screen yesterday and we both are resting better. Thanks for all your prayers. God is in control, what better words can you hear. Connie is a Child of the King, bought and paid for with the shed blood of Jesus Christ. Therefore ALL of the promises in His Word are yes and Amen. That means healing for Connie. Speak to the mountains in your life, give them to God. As much as my heart breaks because I can't hold her hand right now, I am overwhelmed with the peace of God knowing He has this. Thanks everyone.

July 8th pm: Update on Connie… the Dr. called, Connie is still stable with her vitals with medication. Breathing is still relying heavy on the ventilator. The next few days will be crucial for her. They will be bringing her ventilator down to check for the damage that the stroke has caused checking to see if she can cough and swallow. There is a risk because she is relying on the ventilator to breathe. They are concerned that the stroke has affected her ability to be able to cough or swallow.

Pray that she has no complications while they are doing these procedures. And that pneumonia will not set in her lungs. She is still not responding on her left side. Dr. said she has major complications, complicating her overcoming the virus. Thanks for your prayers.

July 9th am: Update on Connie, there were no changes thru the night. Reminds me of how the tides always have to stop flowing in one direction before the tide changes to the opposite directions. Connie has had enough bad news. It is time for the tide to change. There's a miracle in the making. Thanks for all your Prayers and support.

July 9th pm: Update on Connie… today was not a good day. The procedure to back off the ventilator to see what damage the stroke has cause to her being able to swallow, did not reveal the results that we were praying for. When they tried to back it off, Connie's condition would not allow them to complete the process. Connie's oxygen saturation in her blood is very low even with the ventilator. The virus is not letting her process the oxygen that she needs. She has now started running a high fever again. This is not the news we wanted to hear today. But God. Saying that changes everything. Connie's condition may sound bad, we have been here before. There is nothing that my Lord can't handle. We serve a Big God and there is nothing that catches Him by surprise. Thanks for all your prayers and support.

July 10th am: Update on Connie…the doctor's tried another breathing trial last night, PTL Connie passed that one. This means they may be able in a few days to take the ventilator out to evaluate the effects that the stroke has had on her being able to swallow. Her fever is still high. They are treating it to bring it down. Nurse said that Connie is still only responding to commands on her right side. She is resting better this morning. I know Connie is going to be overwhelmed when she sees how our community has been interceding for her. And not only prayers from the community but warriors from all over. Thanks for your continue Prayers. God's hands have been moved. As I said in a earlier post. BUT GOD

July 10th pm: Friday evening update on Connie Ivey…the progress that Connie made last night and this morning she lost this afternoon. With that said, I have to remind myself that Sunday Connie was fighting for her life. And today she is critical but stable. Praise the Lord for the progress that Connie has made this week. Thanks for all your prayers and support and I will leave you with just two more words, words that changes everything. BUT GOD…

July 11th am: Saturday morning update on Connie Ivey..Connie was able to pass another breathing trial her fever has dropped some but still is high. They were able to turn her ventilator down to 55 pct, but she still has no response on her left side. Prayers are working. The most exciting thing that Connie did is when they had the meds cut back to do the breathing trial Connie picked her right hand up and started fanning towards her face. The nurse ask Connie was she hot and she nodded her head yes. This is the first communication that Connie initiated herself. They are in trouble now. They have been giving her commands over and over testing to see where she is at. I think the tide is about to change. I have been married to Connie for 40 plus years Please keep the nurses in your prayers. Great news this morning, PTL, thanks for all you support. And remember whatever you may be facing in your life repeat these two words and it will change your perspective. BUT GOD…

July 11th pm: Saturday afternoon update on Connie Ivey…if you are sitting down you may need to stand up and get ready to do a victory dance. Connie is off the ventilator. They did another breathing trial and were able to remove the ventilator. Right now she is coping ok with the assist of an oxygen tube. PTL let me say that again. That does not need to be abbreviated. PRAISE THE LORD.!!!!!!! Everything else is still the same. Tomorrow they will be checking to see what effects the stroke had on her. God has moved in an awesome way. Thanks for all your prayers. We need to continue to pray specifically that she will be able to swallow. I am so thankful, now give the Lord the Praise and please share this post. I want everyone to see the power of God first hand. And remember BUT GOD changes everything.

July 12th am: Letter to Connie, Connie Ivey: I am writing this to you so you can hopefully and prayerfully be able to read it soon. It has been 18 days since I have been able to hold you. My heart is so heavy and this hurts like nothing I have ever experienced. The last few updates that I have received from the nurses have been so much better. Connie when you see how everyone family, friends and the community and beyond has been calling out your name to the Lord for you. You are going to be so overwhelmed. You are so loved. God has blessed us so much. I remember before we were married and I was shrimping with Capt. Pete on the *Amor* it didn't matter how many days we were gone or what time of day or night we returned back to the dock. There would always be this beautiful brown-eyed girl waiting on the dock waving her arms and jumping with excitement to see me and hold me. I'm telling you, Connie Ivey, I will be there waving my arms and jumping with excitement when they allow me to see you and hold you in my arms again. I love you Connie Ivey, other than

Jesus Christ saving me before we ever got married, YOU are the best thing that has ever happened to me.

July 12th pm: Sunday morning update on Connie Ivey…Connie is still off the ventilator, she is continuing to require less oxygen, she has finally broke the fever this morning. It sounds like the hold that the virus has had on her lungs has finally released. They will soon in the next few days be evaluating the damage from the stroke. She needs to be able to swallow. Thanks again for all your prayers and support. It has given us strength when there was none and encouragement when I was down, God is not though with Connie, BUT GOD…

July 13th: Monday morning update on Connie Ivey. There have not been any major changes since yesterday. Thanks for all your prayers. She needs to be able to swallow. But God…

July 14th: Tuesday morning update on Connie Ivey. Connie is still in ICU she is critical but stable. She is still off the ventilator. There has been little change in the last few days. Still no sign of any movement on her left side and still no sign of her being able to swallow is reported. They are still evaluating the extent of the stroke. Connie is a fighter but most important Connie is a child of the King. And there is nothing impossible with God. Thank you Lord, for Connie's healing. I want to thank each and every one of you for the prayers and support that you have shown. I realize that with the reports that have been coming in, Connie has a hard road ahead of her. BUT GOD!!!

July 15th: Wednesday morning update on Connie Ivey. Not a lot of changes through the night. Thanks for all your prayers.

July 16th: Thursday morning update on Connie Ivey. Connie has taken a step backwards. With the stroke causing her not to be able to swallow or cough it is causing other concerns with her lungs. Thanks for all your prayers and support. I know Connie, when she gets to where she can see all the people that has responded, will be so overwhelmed. Today makes 22-days since I was able to hold her hand and assure her that everything will be ok. I know that even though I can't see her or hold her as I have always promised her I would, God has this. The Holy Spirit is her Comforter, and He is her Healer, her strength and her peace. Connie is a child of the King and that is where I draw my strength. I know that if I never get to look into her big brown eyes again here on this earth, I will see her again. I Love you Connie Ivey, I miss you so much. God is not finished with you. BUT GOD…

July 17th: Friday evening update on Connie Ivey. I was able to see my sweetie today though Zoom. I really appreciate the nurses that made that happen. There are a lot of preparations that they have to do because of the virus. Connie is still in need of a miracle. The stroke was severe which is causing a lot of complications. She still is not showing any movement on her left side or being able to swallow. There is much concern with her lungs. Today when I saw Connie thru Zoom I was hoping to have the same response that I had 10 days ago when her eyes lit up when she saw me. That didn't happen. My heart is so heavy. Pray for healing. Connie's faith will get her though this, for she is in the Lord's hands. I thank each one of you for all your prayers and support, this community has something that a lot of places don't have. That is people like you that put their own needs on hold and intercede for others. There are so many in our small community that needs our prayers that it gets overwhelming. But know that your Prayers don't go unheard. We are drawing support from them. Thanks. #But God…

July 18th: Update on Connie Ivey Saturday evening, 23rd day. Connie is about the same as yesterday. They do have better control of the seizures this afternoon. She is not having them as often. There is still no response on the left side or her showing any sign of being able to swallow. The reports are not what we are wanted to hear. But I choose to believe the report of the Lord. Connie is a child of the King therefore the Promises of God is yes and amen. And that includes her Healing. Thanks for all your prayers and support and Please continue to lift Ray Patty Leazer and Legrand Phelps up in your prayers also. #But God…

July 19th: Update on Connie Ivey Sunday morning 24th day. Connie has been moved to the COVID-19 floor. Everything is about the same. We are still expecting a miracle. Thanks for all your prayers. I thank the Lord for my family, and their strong faith. Now as Connie would want, we are headed to church with our Praise on. Lord show up in a mighty way we need your strength and your peace. God is in Control. #But God…

July 20th: Update on Connie Ivey Monday morning 25th day. No changes through the night; they are keeping her comfortable and she is resting. Thanks for all your prayers and support #But God…

July 21st: Update on Connie Ivey Tuesday, 26th day. No real change in Connie this morning. Still believing in her healing. Thank you everyone that has prayed for Gerald and Connie both. Keep the prayers coming. THANK YOU.

July 22nd: Update on Connie Ivey Wednesday, 27th day. There is not much change in Connie. Dr. is keeping her comfortable and she is resting. The stroke has caused major complications slowing her Healing process. Connie knows the Healer. She has a personal relationship with Him. And He knows her by her name. The Comforter (which is the Holy Ghost) has not left her side. For days when Connie first started battling this virus and she was able to speak, she told the nurse that I have been there the whole time. That is the peace that only God gives. I know and believe that even though Connie is not alert as she was, the Holy Spirit is comforting her and I have to think that in Connie's mind I am right beside her holding her hand as I have for 45 years. I love you Connie. Thanks for all the prayers and support. #But God…

July 23rd: Update on Connie Ivey Thursday, day 28. First I want to say thanks for all the prayers and support though this difficult time. Connie is now under Hospice care. They will be bringing her home tomorrow. I will finally get to hold my sweeties hands. And look into those big brown eyes of hers and tell her how much I love her and have missed her. I can't wait to tell her how this small community and beyond had been interceding for her. I have recently been diagnosed with pneumonia, please pray that I can fight it off so I will not be hospitalized. Connie needs me these next few days and I need her. Connie will soon receive her Healing. Again thanks and please continue to lift the different ones in our small community and beyond up in Prayers. Prayers move the hand of God. This will be my last post for a few days. Thanks.

July 25ᵗʰ: Update on Connie Ivey and Gerald Ivey. This morning I feel like I finally made the turn on the double pneumonia. It is amazing how fast things change when your sweetie is beside you holding hands. Thank you for all your prayers and support. There is a miracle in the making. The miracles are still happening as time revolves. Please continue to lift each other up in prayers; there are many in our small communities that need our continuing prayers. Again thanks, Gerald.

July 29ᵗʰ: Last Update for Connie Ivey Wednesday July 29ᵗʰ. At 7:09 this morning Connie received her Healing. She has been made whole. I want to thank each one of you that have been lifting Connie and me up in your prayers. Not only did I get to bring my big brown-eyed girl home, I was able to hold her hand and talk to her. And tell her the way this community and beyond has been praying for her. Your prayers were answered, Connie has received the ultimate Healing, and she is now walking on the streets of gold, hand and hand with Jesus. I will be fine, this is not the last time I will see her. Please continue to pray for the different needs in this small community. There are many needs. As we have witnessed with Connie, Prayers Work. #But God…

July 29th: From Will, Connie Ivey (Momma) received her healing in the highest way this morning. Thank you all for the continued prayers, love and support for our family.

I am so ever grateful for having such an amazing Mama, she not only taught Gerik and myself how to walk tall, set the standard high, not lower our standards just because it's the easy way out, walk close with The Lord, and all the other life lessons but she also walked the walk and showed us how to do the same. She was a Beautiful Amazing Woman.

She helped so many people. I thank God that he chose me to be a part of her life.

Aug. 1st: Update on Connie Ivey Connie Ivey Memorial

Family Night: Friday (7/31/20), 6-8 at White Funeral Home in Bolivia, NC.

Funeral: Saturday (8/1/20), 11:00 at Harvest Fellowship IPHC in Shallotte. Graveside to follow at Union Chapel in Supply. Will be limited space at the church; however, we are opening the fellowship hall for additional seating. We will also be posting Facebook live of the service.

Aug. 1ˢᵗ: From Gerik, I just want to take a minute and brag on this woman I call mama. She was a kind and loving woman, she had a big heart for everyone no matter who you were. At the same time she did not put up with nonsense from anyone and would tell you like it was. She loved God with all her heart and was always faithful even in the many hard times she had. She loved my daddy, Gerald Ivey, with all her heart and he loved her just as much. She helped to set a strong foundation for my brother, Will Ivey, and I She loved us unconditionally and was always there whether we needed uplifting or to be set straight.

190

Connie Ivey had a big impact on everyone she spent any amount of time with and was a special woman and always will be in my heart. We love you and will definitely miss you, but we know you are rejoicing in heaven and you will always be with us. Gone from here but never forgotten. Mama, thank you for being a bright light in our lives and thank you for being a strong woman of God.

Aug.14th: I would like to take this time to say thanks for all the acts of kindness that each one of you has shown me and my family through this difficult time. We were so overwhelmed by the way you reached out to us, whether you sent flowers, food, gifts, cards, phone call or your prayers, we greatly appreciated it. I have tried to send out thank you cards to each one, unfortunately I no longer have Connie here to remind me who did what so I would not forget anyone. Please if you have sent any act of kindness know that I and my family want to say thanks. May God bless you many times over. Please continue to remember us in your prayers. I am still struggling with pneumonia in both lungs hopefully the next set of X-rays will show progress. Again thanks.

Aug. 29th: One month ago at 7:09 am Connie took her last breath here on this Earth. She is now rejoicing with many loved ones that have gone on before her. Two weeks after Connie went home to be with the Lord, Ronnie her brother (Skins) joined her. I know they are walking hand and hand together on the streets of Gold. I will miss her but she would not come back for anything. I promised Connie that I would be okay. I have not lived up to that promise too well. This is hard. You see on July 29th at 7:09 in the morning, my life changed forever; half of me died that day. The love of my life is gone. I know my Lord and Savior will see me through this. He is my Peace, my strength, and my Comforter. I have never felt such pain in my life. Everywhere I look I see memories of Connie. We had so many great memories together but the little things that we did that no one else would understand, like it might have been a smile, a look, some crazy jester or a gentle touch, is now gone. Realization is setting in. I am so thankful for my family, I know they are going through pain also as they lost their mama, their Nana and their friend. But they have been so strong and supportive. I am so blessed. We will be fine. We will lean on each other and draw strength from our Lord. I know that I will continue to have my moments. (Pastor said that is normal) I will never forget that God joined Connie and me together for over 40 yrs. We had a beautiful marriage and our love for each other was never questioned. Our love for Christ never wavered. We will see each other again. If you still have your spouse hold them a little tighter, spend as much time with them as you can. Continue to share those little jester's, life changes very quickly. Connie's legacy will live on through me, her children, grandchildren and those that she touched throughout her life. Thanks for all your prayers and support during these tough times, continue to pray for the needs of our community and our nation. God Bless each one of you.

November 3: Happy birthday Connie Ivey. Today, Nov. 3rd, you would have turned 59 years old We were looking forward to growing old together. That's not going to happen. I remember holding your hand when you turned 13 years old at church. We were so young and happy. Our love for each other was so solid. We grew up together. Wow, so many memories. God blessed me with a wonderful wife, a friend, mother of my children, my soul mate. Today they are supposed to set our headstone. I know that you would like what I picked out, Connie. In the center there is the picture of the last time we held hands. I know when you released my hand for the last time, you were reaching up to take Jesus' hand. I can't help but remember the chorus to that song that you sung so many times at Union Chapel. *What a day that will be When my Jesus I shall see When I look upon His face. The One who saved me by His grace. When He takes me by the hand and leads me to the Promised Land what a day, glorious day that will be.* That day came for you July 29th. I will always remember God granted me true love for over 40 years. I will miss you but I will see you again. I love you.

Dec, 24th: Christmas will never be the same, I miss you so much Connie Ivey, So many great memories, Christmas was always your favorite time of the year. God blessed us so much. You will never be forgotten Connie, you touched so many lives. My heart is so broken. Lord, you are my strength. You are my Comforter. I need your peace. Help me though this journey. Help me though the next minute. I feel so lost.

January 29th, 2021: It is hard to believe that it has been 6-months since the Love of my life crossed over to Heaven. It still seems like it was yesterday that I was holding your hand, Connie Ivey. I keep thinking what could I have done different, how could I avoided this from happening. It was out of my control Connie. I tried so hard but I couldn't fix it this time baby. I loved you so much. But God had a different plan for you. I know and I have to keep reminding myself that you have found true happiness and complete healing. That you are now walking on the streets of glory. I know that I will see you again. But the pain and the lost that I feel is so unbearable at times. I miss you so much everyday Connie. I thank the Lord every day for the memories of the last 45 years that I got to share with you. You were such a remarkable woman, such a loving wife. And I know that I can speak for Will Ivey and Gerik N Rachel Ivey that you were an awesome momma. You were so anointed. You touched so many lives. You changed mine. We were so blessed. I miss you so much. I will be ok Connie. I will continue to draw my strength from my Lord and Savior. He is my strength my comforter and my peace. I will always love you and miss you. Only God can fill the emptiness that I now have.

Feb. 13th: Tomorrow will be the first Valentine's Day in 44 years that I will not be able to show the love of my life, Connie Ivey, how much I love her. I am so thankful that we showed each other every day, as I sit here and stare at her pictures and look back at the memories we made together. My heart is so broken. I miss Connie so much. I know that God blessed me with the most beautiful woman and friend. She showed me every day how much she loved me. I am so thankful for the memories that we made though out our lifetime together. Happy Valentine's Day, Connie you are and will always be MY VALENTINE.

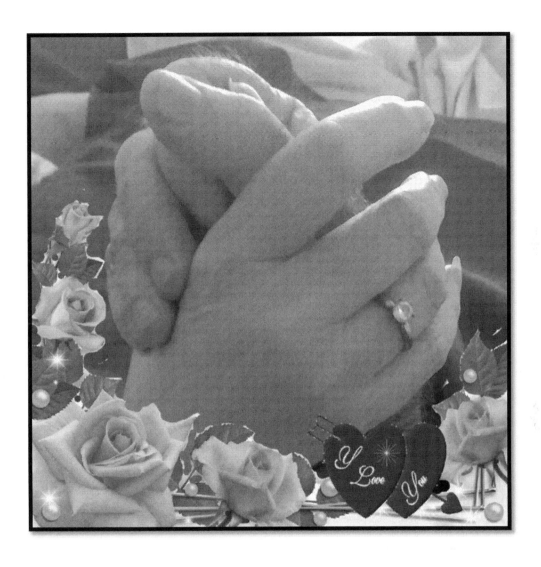

The last physical contact of two partners in life, Connie and Gerald.

1 Corinthians 13:13 - So now faith, hope, and love abide, these three; but the greatest of these is love.

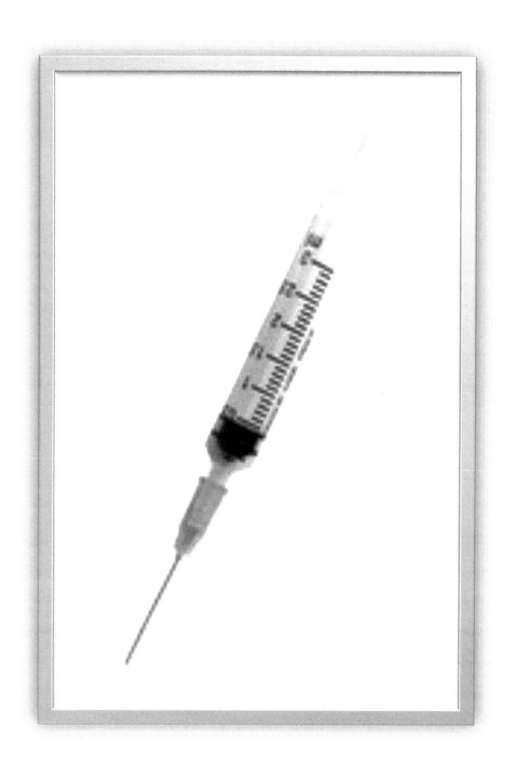

194

Chapter 8

Vaccinations and Variants Arrived

It is unclear whether this disease will continue in the present form and frequency until summer arrives, or will continue through the fall of 2021. At one point, it was suggested that it would wind down by fall of 2020. That did not happen. The next goal was perhaps fall of 2021. Since it is the first time this virus has hit the world, too many unknowns remain.

One must remember, that among all the death and sickness, are so many instances of positive people, heroic actions, and immeasurable love has been shared with others through actions and contacts. These have occurred throughout the globe, country, county and home town of each of us. Everyone has their own story to share. The reader is encouraged to document their own experiences in Chapter 10 before they begin to fade from memory.

Vaccines

One of the miracles being experienced in the spring of 2021 is the availability of the COVID vaccine. By March 2021, the United States had surpassed 500 thousand deaths. At the same time, a milestone of over 3 million people was vaccinated.

Total vaccines distributed: 4,765,300. Total Administered: 3,813,176.

A tested, safe and effective vaccine became available in early spring of 2021, but supplies were limited at first. Independent state and federal public health advisory committees determined that the best way to fight COVID-19 was to start first with vaccinations for those most at risk, reaching more people as the vaccine supply increases from January to June. People were encouraged to keep practicing the 3 Ws —wear a mask, wait six feet apart, wash your hands—until everyone had a chance to vaccinate.

By Easter 2021, everyone wanted to know which of the three vaccines in the United States, was the best, with some waiting for the Johnson and Johnson because it only involved one vaccination instead of two. Lingering questions remain and new ones popped up. How long are you contagious with the virus? What about flying? What is the survival rate? Can you die from a vaccine? Are you a carrier if you have a vaccine? Can you still get it if you are vaccinated? Is the compound in the vaccine harmful in other ways?

The CDC said the vaccines were tested, safe and effective against COVID-19. They passed clinical trials and in this Covid emergency but have not yet been approved by the

Federal Drug Administration. However in this emergency situation, the FDA allowed the use of the vaccines for individuals 16 years of age and older. There are three safe vaccines provided by Pfizer, Moderna and Johnson & Johnson by June 2021.

Each state had their computer dashboard to follow the state guidelines laid out by the Governor. Vaccines were also issued based upon state data; such as population, number testing positive, etc. Each state varies slightly in their processes and to whom the vaccines are available. The CDC had updated information on COVID-19 vaccines, including recommendations processes, differences about the different types, their benefits, safety data, and frequently asked questions.

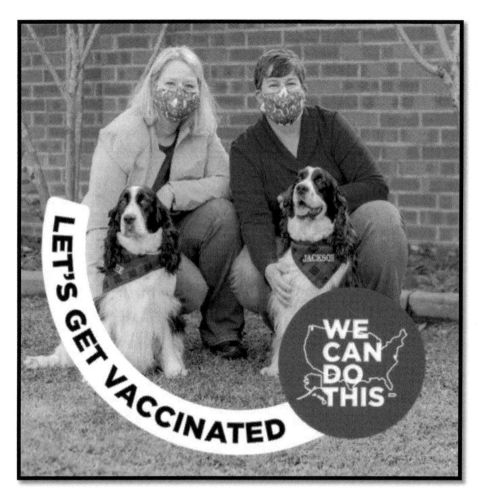

Figure 68 Leona Walfield and Leigh Sauls.

Leona Walfield, BS, MBA,

Leigh Sauls, BSN, CRNA, (Certified Registered Nurse Anesthetist)

with their Springer spaniels:

Annie, 4

and

Jackson, 6;

show their support for the Covid vaccination. Many others on social media also posted their support of vaccinations encouraging everyone to get it as soon as offered.

Understanding the Vaccine Distribution Phases

Many people were afraid of getting the vaccine and many others waited anxiously for their "group" to be allowed to receive the vaccine. Most states followed the CDC guidelines and divided their populations into five groups. Getting the vaccine was a challenge for many.

An example of the assigned groups can be demonstrated by the North Carolina's Active Vaccine Groups in March of 2021 and include: Group 1, 2, 3, and 4.

Group 1: Health care workers with in-person patient contact; long-term care staff and residents—people in skilled nursing facilities, adult care homes and continuing care retirement communities.

Group 2: Anyone 65 years or older, regardless of health status or living situation.

Group 3: Frontline essential workers who are in sectors essential to the functioning of society and who are at substantially higher risk for exposure to COVID-19.

Group 4: People with high-risk medical conditions, people experiencing homelessness, and incarcerated people who have not been vaccinated. Ages 16-64 with higher risk medical conditions and additional congregate settings.

The NCDHHS announced plans for how the state could move to *Group 4* for COVID-19 vaccines. The following individuals from Group 4 became eligible to schedule and receive vaccines on Wednesday, April 7: Essential workers not yet vaccinated and other people in close group living settings.

Group 5: Included everyone else not yet eligible in Group 1-4.

Vaccine Issues

Individuals who have certain medical problems or are pregnant (or nursing) are not encouraged to get the vaccine. Individuals who have any allergies a fever, a bleeding disorder or on blood thinner or have a compromised immune system are not candidates for the vaccines at this time.

According to the CDC, "All the COVID-19 vaccines give the cells in your body the instructions to make a protein that safely teaches your body how to make antibodies (germ-fighting cells) to fight the real COVID-19. Your body naturally destroys the instructions and gets rid of them. None of the vaccine ingredients remain in your system, nor do they alter any DNA in your body. The three COVID-19 vaccines currently available in the United States do not contain eggs, preservatives, fetal tissue, stem cells, mercury or latex."

Pfizer-BioNTech COVID-19 vaccine ingredients: The Pfizer-BioNTech COVID-19 Vaccine includes the following ingredients: mRNA, lipids ((4-hydroxybutyl) azanediyl) bis (hexane-6,1-diyl) bis (2-hexyldecanoate), 2 [(polyethylene glycol)-2000]-N,Nditetradecylacetamide, 1,2-Distearoyl-sn-glycero-3- phosphocholine, and cholesterol), potassium chloride, monobasic potassium phosphate, sodium chloride, dibasic sodium phosphate dihydrate, and sucrose. The Pfizer vaccine is given in the arm muscle in two doses; three weeks apart. Pfizer was made by ingredients from New York and Germany.

Moderna COVID-19 vaccine ingredients: messenger ribonucleic acid (mRNA), lipids (SM-102, polyethylene glycol [PEG] 2000 dimyristoyl glycerol [DMG], cholesterol, and 1,2-distearoyl-sn-glycero-3-phosphocholine [DSPC]), tromethamine, tromethamine hydrochloride, acetic acid, sodium acetate trihydrate, and sucrose. The Moderna vaccine is given in two doses in the arm, one month apart. Moderna is home-based in Texas and Massachusettes, USA.

Johnson & Johnson COVID-19 vaccine, called the Janssen Vaccine, ingredients include: recombinant, replication-incompetent adenovirus type 26 expressing the SARS-CoV-2 spike protein, citric acid monohydrate, trisodium citrate dihydrate, ethanol, 2-hydroxypropyl-β-cyclodextrin (HBCD), polysorbate-80, sodium chloride. This vaccine is given one time only in the arm muscle. It is manufactured in Pennsylvania by the Janssen Pharmaceutical Company, a part of Johnson and Johnson.

Side Effects of the Vaccines

Side effect of the vaccines included: injection site pain, tiredness, headache, muscle pain, chills, joint pain, fever, injection site swelling, injection site redness, nausea, feeling unwell, swollen lymph nodes (lymphadenopathy), non-severe allergic reactions such as rash, itching, hives, or swelling of the face, and severe allergic reactions.

Some people may also have experienced severe allergic reactions such as difficulty breathing, swelling of your face and throat. fast heartbeat, bad rash all over your body, and dizziness and weakness. Of course, with those severe reactions, individuals needed to go to the hospital for care.

Many remained confused…to vaccinate or not. However some received positive benefits after suffering from some apparent Covid symptoms for over a year. Symptoms like headaches, shortness of breath, extreme fatigue and problems with smell, among other symptoms simply disappeared after getting the Covid vaccine.[76]

Some Catholics were confused as to whether it was morally acceptable to get the vaccine, especially the Johnson and Johnson vaccine due to reports that it included a cell line from an abortion in its production.   Later, it was determined that it was acceptable if

---

[76]Health News from NPR. The Corona Crisis. March 31 2021   https://www.npr.org/sections/health-shots/2021/03/31/982799452/mysterious-ailment-mysterious-relief-vaccines-help-some-covid-long-haulers

the only vaccine available. Other reports denied the use of cells from abortion. This matter remains unclear to many.

Others within the reproductive ages are hesitant to get the vaccine due to possible infertility. The last argument I've heard from people choosing to wait to get the vaccine assumes the vaccine could cause infertility in women.

This theory may have originated from a German doctor. He was concerned about an ingredient of the vaccine: a protein called syncytin-1. The syncytin-1 protein has similar genetic construction as found within COVID-19, but it is also a vital component in the make-up of the placenta in most mammals. He was concerned that this protein might cause the body to fight the placenta when she becomes pregnant causing infertility.

Other developers, while agreeing the syncytin-1 was similar to human placenta, it was not identical and did not believe it might cause infertility.

The doctors at the University of Alabama at Birmingham echo others who recommend getting the vaccine, even if pregnancy plans are in the woman's near future. They have published that it is safer to get the vaccine than not, in this circumstance.[77]

Another study by Pfizer indicated the vaccine in animal studies did not cause harmful effects on ability to conceive a baby. This truly frightened parents trying to decide whether their younger children, aged 16 and up should even get the vaccine. Would it hurt their chances of having children in the future? No one knew. By June 8th 2021, 12 year olds were eligible and encouraged to get the vaccine. News reports featured parents afraid of having their children vaccinated.

Blood Clots

Then the Johnson and Johnson vaccine showed causation to blood clots in a very small number of those receiving the vaccines. Administration of this particular vaccine was halted for a couple of weeks until doctors recommended to re-start the offering of this vaccine citing the benefits far outweigh the possible side affect, even though deaths were the result. Primarily this was with females but a male in California also experienced a blood clot in his leg.

Scientific American reported that there was only one in a million probability of getting a blood clot due to the vaccine according to Wilber Chen, infectious disease

---

[77] Koplon, Savannah. *Addressing fertility questions and concerns with the COVID-19 vaccine.* University of Alabama News. February 22, 2021.

physician-scientist. [78]   Scientific American Editor's Note: *"At the ACIP (Advisory Committee on Immunization Practices) meeting on April 23, Tom Shimabukuro of the CDC's COVID-19 Vaccine Task Force reported that as of April 21 there have been a total of 15 confirmed cases of this blood clotting condition among nearly eight million doses administered. All of the cases were in women, and the highest risk was among women ages 30 to 39, among whom the rate was 11.8 per million."*

As of April 5, 2021, the following was reported by the Centers for Disease Control:

Cases of Covid in US Last 30 Days: 30,492,334

Total Vaccines Administered: 165,053,746

Total Deaths in US: 553,681

The Variants Emerged

A variant of the Covid virus emerged in early 2021 and by April there were at least five currently known in the United States. The idea of virus variants began to become the focus, along with "Did you get your vaccination yet?"

The CDC grouped these variants by:

VOI: Variant of Interest, "A variant with specific genetic markers that have been associated with changes to receptor binding, reduced neutralization by antibodies generated against previous infection or vaccination, reduced efficacy of treatments, potential diagnostic impact, or predicted increase in transmissibility or disease severity."[79]

VOC: Variant of Concern, "A variant for which there is evidence of an increase in transmissibility, more severe disease (increased hospitalizations or deaths), significant reduction in neutralization by antibodies generated during previous infection or vaccination, reduced effectiveness of treatments or vaccines, or diagnostic detection failures."[80]

---

[78] Daley, Jim. Scientific American. Blood Clots and the Johnson & Johnson Vaccine: What We Know So Far Infectious disease physician-scientist Wilbur Chen discusses the rare cases of blood clots linked to the immunization.   https://www.scientificamerican.com/article/blood-clots-and-the-johnson-johnson-vaccine-what-we-know-so-far/. April 23, 2021.
[79] Centers for Disease Control. SARS-CoV-2 Variant Classifications and Definitions. March 24, 2021.
  https://www.cdc.gov/coronavirus/2019-ncov/cases-updates/variant-surveillance/variant-info.html#Interest
[80] IBID.

VOHC: Variant of High Consequence, "A variant of high consequence has clear evidence that prevention measures or medical countermeasures (MCMs) have significantly reduced effectiveness relative to previously circulating variants."[81]

The specific **variants** known to be in the United States included:

B.1.1.7: This variant was first identified in the US in December 2020. It was initially detected in the UK.

B.1.351: This variant was first identified in the US at the end of January 2021. It was initially detected in South Africa in December 2020.

P.1: This variant was first detected in the US in January 2021. P.1 was initially identified in travelers from Brazil, who were tested during routine screening at an airport in Japan, in early January.

B.1.427 and B.1.429: These two variants were first identified in California in February 2021 and were classified as VOCs in March 2021.

On April 5th, 2021, the following statistic were posted by the CDC:

Variant	Reported Cases in US	Number of Jurisdictions Reporting
B.1.1.7	12,505	51
B.1.351	323	31
P.1	224	22

The following states documented cases (if any) according to the CDC:

State	filter	Cases
AL	Variant B.1.1.7	105
AK	Variant B.1.1.7	3
AS	Variant B.1.1.7	0
AZ	Variant B.1.1.7	95
AR	Variant B.1.1.7	7
CA	Variant B.1.1.7	822

---

[81] IBID.

CO	Variant B.1.1.7	894
CT	Variant B.1.1.7	379
District of Columbia	Variant B.1.1.7	40
DE	Variant B.1.1.7	17
FL	Variant B.1.1.7	2351
GA	Variant B.1.1.7	592
GU	Variant B.1.1.7	0
HI	Variant B.1.1.7	13
ID	Variant B.1.1.7	30
IL	Variant B.1.1.7	218
IN	Variant B.1.1.7	137
IA	Variant B.1.1.7	89
KS	Variant B.1.1.7	27
KY	Variant B.1.1.7	64
LA	Variant B.1.1.7	51
ME	Variant B.1.1.7	15
MH	Variant B.1.1.7	0
MD	Variant B.1.1.7	611
MA	Variant B.1.1.7	712
MI	Variant B.1.1.7	1237
FM	Variant B.1.1.7	0
MN	Variant B.1.1.7	526
MS	Variant B.1.1.7	42
MO	Variant B.1.1.7	16
MT	Variant B.1.1.7	8
NE	Variant B.1.1.7	51
NV	Variant B.1.1.7	62

NH	Variant B.1.1.7	101
NJ	Variant B.1.1.7	389
NM	Variant B.1.1.7	21
NY	Variant B.1.1.7	136
NC	Variant B.1.1.7	178
ND	Variant B.1.1.7	7
MP	Variant B.1.1.7	0
OH	Variant B.1.1.7	398
OK	Variant B.1.1.7	0
OR	Variant B.1.1.7	18
PW	Variant B.1.1.7	0
PA	Variant B.1.1.7	431
PR	Variant B.1.1.7	1
RI	Variant B.1.1.7	7
SC	Variant B.1.1.7	86
SD	Variant B.1.1.7	14
TN	Variant B.1.1.7	318
TX	Variant B.1.1.7	414
UT	Variant B.1.1.7	207
VT	Variant B.1.1.7	12
VI	Variant B.1.1.7	0
VA	Variant B.1.1.7	190
WA	Variant B.1.1.7	223
WV	Variant B.1.1.7	53
WI	Variant B.1.1.7	78
WY	Variant B.1.1.7	9
AL	Variant P.1	0

AK	Variant P.1	5
AS	Variant P.1	0
AZ	Variant P.1	5
AR	Variant P.1	0
CA	Variant P.1	33
CO	Variant P.1	0
CT	Variant P.1	2
District of Columbia	Variant P.1	0
DE	Variant P.1	0
FL	Variant P.1	55
GA	Variant P.1	1
GU	Variant P.1	0
HI	Variant P.1	0
ID	Variant P.1	0
IL	Variant P.1	19
IN	Variant P.1	1
IA	Variant P.1	0
KS	Variant P.1	0
KY	Variant P.1	0
LA	Variant P.1	0
ME	Variant P.1	1
MH	Variant P.1	0
MD	Variant P.1	1
MA	Variant P.1	58
MI	Variant P.1	0
FM	Variant P.1	0
MN	Variant P.1	2

MS	Variant P.1	0
MO	Variant P.1	0
MT	Variant P.1	0
NE	Variant P.1	2
NV	Variant P.1	0
NH	Variant P.1	0
NJ	Variant P.1	3
NM	Variant P.1	0
NY	Variant P.1	0
NC	Variant P.1	0
ND	Variant P.1	0
MP	Variant P.1	0
OH	Variant P.1	10
OK	Variant P.1	1
OR	Variant P.1	1
PW	Variant P.1	0
PA	Variant P.1	0
PR	Variant P.1	0
RI	Variant P.1	0
SC	Variant P.1	0
SD	Variant P.1	0
TN	Variant P.1	4
TX	Variant P.1	3
UT	Variant P.1	3
VT	Variant P.1	0
VI	Variant P.1	0
VA	Variant P.1	0

WA	Variant P.1	13
WV	Variant P.1	0
WI	Variant P.1	1
WY	Variant P.1	0
AL	Variant B.1.351	1
AK	Variant B.1.351	0
AS	Variant B.1.351	0
AZ	Variant B.1.351	0
AR	Variant B.1.351	0
CA	Variant B.1.351	10
CO	Variant B.1.351	23
CT	Variant B.1.351	7
District of Columbia	Variant B.1.351	2
DE	Variant B.1.351	1
FL	Variant B.1.351	16
GA	Variant B.1.351	22
GU	Variant B.1.351	0
HI	Variant B.1.351	5
ID	Variant B.1.351	2
IL	Variant B.1.351	3
IN	Variant B.1.351	2
IA	Variant B.1.351	0
KS	Variant B.1.351	0
KY	Variant B.1.351	0
LA	Variant B.1.351	0
ME	Variant B.1.351	4
MH	Variant B.1.351	0

MD	Variant B.1.351	39
MA	Variant B.1.351	12
MI	Variant B.1.351	5
FM	Variant B.1.351	0
MN	Variant B.1.351	8
MS	Variant B.1.351	1
MO	Variant B.1.351	0
MT	Variant B.1.351	0
NE	Variant B.1.351	0
NV	Variant B.1.351	1
NH	Variant B.1.351	0
NJ	Variant B.1.351	1
NM	Variant B.1.351	0
NY	Variant B.1.351	1
NC	Variant B.1.351	29
ND	Variant B.1.351	0
MP	Variant B.1.351	0
OH	Variant B.1.351	3
OK	Variant B.1.351	0
OR	Variant B.1.351	0
PW	Variant B.1.351	0
PA	Variant B.1.351	3
PR	Variant B.1.351	0
RI	Variant B.1.351	0
SC	Variant B.1.351	68
SD	Variant B.1.351	1
TN	Variant B.1.351	1

TX	Variant B.1.351	3
UT	Variant B.1.351	0
VT	Variant B.1.351	0
VI	Variant B.1.351	0
VA	Variant B.1.351	30
WA	Variant B.1.351	17
WV	Variant B.1.351	0
WI	Variant B.1.351	2
WY	Variant B.1.351	0

Globally, the mutations have spread and continue to mutate creating more variations of the virus. Some are deemed more deadly; others less deadly than COVID-19. These new variations continue to emerge. Scientists are continuing to research these mutations and trying to determine the effectiveness of the current vaccines on these new strains. All health agencies, world-wide are watching and documenting these changes; sometimes as many as 17 mutations off of one base virus. Time will tell the complete story.

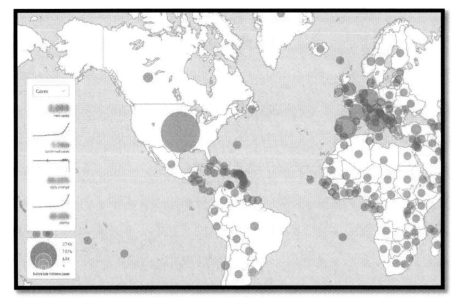

As of **29 April 2021**, a total of **968,452,196 vaccine doses** have been administered.

Around the globe, the World Health Organization documented the following numbers on April 29, 2021:

Situation by WHO Region

Americas	61,630,065 confirmed cases and 1,499,741 confirmed deaths.
Europe	51,419,852 confirmed cases and 1,075,460 confirmed deaths.

	Confirmed Cases	Confirmed Deaths
South-East Asia	21,444,420	268,598
Eastern Mediterranean	9,017,147	180,906
Africa	3,296,256	82,431
Western Pacific	2,408,498	36,879

By country according to the WHO: Number of deaths (listed in order of greatest number of *confirmed cases* but not necessarily number of deaths.

Country		Deaths
United States of America		567,971
Brazil		639
Mexico		215,547
India		204,832
United Kingdom		127,480
Italy		120,256
Russia Federation		109,731
France		103,234
Germany		82,544
Spain		77,943
Columbia		72,235
Iran		70,966
Turkey		39,398
Argentina		62,599
Columbia		72,235
Poland		67,073
Ukraine		43,778
Peru		60,416
Indonesia		45,116
Czechia		29,213
South Africa		54,285

Country		Deaths
Netherlands		17,104
Canada		24,065
Chili		26,073
Iraq		15,392
Romania		27,833
Country		**Deaths**
Philippines		17,031
Belgium		27,140
Sweden		14,000
Israel		6,361
Portugal		16,973
Pakistan		17,530
Hungary		27,358
Bangladesh		11,305
Jordan		8,754
Serbia		6,312
Switzerland		9,945
Austria		9,903
Japan		10,107
Lebanon		7,224
United Arab Emerites		1,580
Morocco		9,015
Saudi Arabia		6,935
Bulgaria		16,278
Malaysia		1,477
Slovakia		11,647
Ecuador		18,470
Kazakhstan		4,345
Panama		6,216
Belarus		2,522
Greece		10,242
Coratia		7,040
Occupied Palestinia		3,474
Azerbaijan		4,461
Nepal		3,211
Georgia		4,095
Tunisia		10,563
Bolivia (Plurinational State of)		12,885
Paraguay		6,094
Nepal		3,211
Georgia		4,095
Kuwait		1,546
Dominican Republic		3,467
Ethiopia		3,639
Republic of Moldova		5,780
Denmark		2,481

Ireland		4,896	
Lithuania		3,916	
Costa Rica		3,186	
Slovenia		4,530	
Egypt		13,219	
Guatemala		7,478	
Armenia		4,087	
Honduras		5,212	
Qatar		445	
Bosnia and Herzegovina		8,464	
Venezuela (Bolivarian Republic of) 2,082		2,082	
Oman		2,001	
Uruguay		2,452	
Libya		3,019	
Bahrain		632	
Nigeria		2,063	
Kenya		2,688	
North Macedonia		4,772	
Myanmar		3,209	
Albania		2,386	
Republic of Korea		1,825	
Latvia		2,118	
Norway		753	
Sri Lanka		661	
Kosovo		2,143	
Cuba		614	
China		4,857	
Montenegro		1,478	
Kyrgyzstan		1,598	
Ghana		779	
Zambia		1,249	
Uzbekistan		647	
Finland		913	
Mozambique		814	
El Salvador		2,117	
Luxembourg		792	
Cameroon		991	
Cyprus		306	
Slovenia		4,530	
Egypt		13,219	
Guatemala		7,478	
Armenia		4,087	
Honduras		5,212	
Qatar		445	

Bosnia and Herzegovina		8,464
Venezuela (Bolivarian Republic of) 2,082		2,082
Oman		2,001
Uruguay		2,452
Libya		3,019
Bahrain		632
Nigeria		2,063
Kenya		2,688
North Macedonia		4,772
Myanmar		3,209
Albania		2,386
Puerto Rico		2,285
Estonia		1,148
Algeria		3,234
Republic of Korea		1,825
Latvia		2,118
Norway		753
Thailand		188
Singapore		30
Afghanistan		2,618
Namibia		638
Botswana		702
Côte d'Ivoire		285
Jamaica		770
Uganda		341
Senegal		1,107
Zimbabwe		1,565
Madagascar		631
Malawi		1,147
Sudan		2,349
Mongolia		97
Malta		413
Democratic Republic of the Congo		763
Australia		910
Maldives		72
Angola		591
Rwanda		332
Cabo Verde		213
Gabon		138
Syrian Arab Republic		1,572
Guinea		141
Réunion		148
Mayotte		170
French Guiana		100

		141
French Polynesia		141
Eswatini		671
Mauritania		455
Somalia		713
Mali		477
Guadeloupe		211
Tajikistan		91
Burkina Faso		157
Andorra		125
Turkmenistan		0

No cases - Tonga Tokelau Saint Helena Pitcairn Islands
Palau Niue Nauru Micronesia (Federated States of)
Kiribati Democratic People's Republic of Korea
Cook Islands American Samoa

Statistics for the U. S. on April 29, 2021

State	7-day Average Cases	7-day Average Deaths	Total Cases	Total Deaths
Alabama	388	10	527,083	10,879
Alaska	160	2	65,100	341
Arizona	710	12	860,773	17,282
Arkansas	175	3	335,289	5,726
California	1,764	55	3,634,778	60,273
Colorado	1,698	8	506,405	6,273
Connecticut	709	8	337,961	8,080
Delaware	264	3	103,844	1,622

State	7-day Average Cases	7-day Average Deaths	Total Cases	Total Deaths
District of Columbia	85	1	47,533	1,104
Florida	5,456	59	2,222,546	35,030
Georgia	908	38	877,816	20,098
Hawaii	83	1	32,110	482
Idaho	216	2	187,269	2,045
Illinois	2,700	28	1,328,454	24,211
Indiana	995	9	721,145	13,312
Iowa	374	5	363,929	5,930
Kansas	232	2	308,510	4,978
Kentucky	527	16	442,618	6,485
Louisiana	421	7	457,326	10,367
Maine	318	1	60,691	778
Maryland	958	14	445,493	8,637
Massachusetts	1,203	11	643,742	17,578
Michigan	4,709	67	928,407	18,600
Minnesota	1,654	10	572,025	7,113
Mississippi	239	4	311,493	7,193

State	7-day Average Cases	7-day Average Deaths	Total Cases	Total Deaths
Missouri	630	7	584,069	8,738
Montana	136	1	108,489	1,567
Nebraska	236	2	217,702	2,236
Nevada	389	9	314,475	5,448
New Hampshire	287	3	94,405	1,296
New Jersey	877	34	993,486	25,509
New Mexico	205	4	197,218	4,051
New York	3,862	53	2,024,553	51,829
North Carolina	1,858	20	965,546	12,619
North Dakota	134	0	107,154	1,486
Ohio	1,513	22	1,068,985	19,188
Oklahoma	236	10	447,299	6,788
Oregon	826	3	182,916	2,490
Pennsylvania	3,515	43	1,143,076	26,129
Rhode Island	279	1	147,601	2,668
South Carolina	753	15	576,639	9,472
South Dakota	126	1	122,398	1,962

State	7-day Average Cases	7-day Average Deaths	Total Cases	Total Deaths
Tennessee	1,078	9	845,380	12,171
Texas	3,222	49	2,876,542	49,077
Utah	380	2	396,522	2,190
Vermont	69	0	22,723	246
Virginia	1,078	14	657,154	10,735
Washington	1,419	7	400,149	5,474
West Virginia	345	-18	152,301	2,673
Wisconsin	718	12	658,696	6,807
Wyoming	69	0	57,999	707

Statistics are for each state in the United States as of April 29, 2021:

TOTAL CASES	32,031,068	+53,051 New Cases
CASES IN LAST 7 DAYS	367,697	
TOTAL DEATHS	571,297	+876 New Deaths

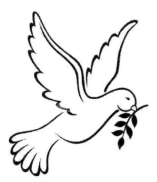

NEW CASES PER DAY

In the United States, there were 57,491 newly reported COVID-19 cases and 928 newly reported COVID-deaths on April 28, 2021. COVID lives on.

Note: For more on how USA Facts collects coronavirus data, read this detailed methodology and sources page.

Chapter 9

What Next?

Scott Atlas, at the Hoover Institution at Stanford University, previously serving as a professor and Chief of Neuroradiology at Stanford University Medical Center pretty well summed up what many of us have been feeling. He said, "The Covid pandemic has been a tragedy, no doubt. But it has exposed **profound issues in America** that threaten the principles of freedom and order that we Americans often take for granted. First, I have been shocked at the unprecedented exertion of power by the government since last March—issuing unilateral decrees, ordering the closure of businesses churches and schools restricting person movement, mandating behavior, and suspending indefinitely basic freedoms. Second, I was and remain stunned—almost frightened—at the acquiescence of the American people to such destructive, arbitrary, and wholly unscientific rules restrictions, and mandates."

Owners of **large tech media companies** censoring individuals and the political influences on science and our society affected us all. The pandemic literally paralyzed our country; and no doubt many other countries as well. Mandates limited our mobility while the number of cases continuing to escalate. Businesses closed, even those who had been in existence for a lifetime as they could no longer pay the bills while the business was prohibited from operating at normal pace. Millions of Americans had difficulty keeping up with living expenses and their mortgage. It appeared that all the mitigating factors trying to lessen the impact of the virus was minimal at best according to numerous studies, including the one at Stanford University infectious disease epidemiologists.

The **impacts of the lockdowns and mandates** may have even been harmful. Closing schools may be producing poor education, dropouts, social isolation and student suicidal thoughts. The costs of those lockdowns for extensive periods of time, is a sad memory for some whose teens committed suicide. In addition, people staying away from medical care and routine medical screenings have a result of millions of new cancers pediatric illnesses, heart attack and strokes. The CDC has reported four times as many cases of depression, anxiety and double the suicidal ideations, particularly among young adults. The American Medical Association reported increased drug overdoses and suicides. Child abuse and domestic abuse increased.

Even some governors, like Florida Governor Ron DeSantis said lockdowns were a huge mistake. Everyone wanted to mitigate the damages but one year later, using a 15-day lockdown, then a 30 day lockdown, and then long-term lockdowns, masks and shutdowns of businesses, did not work. While some states were more lenient than others, it did not stop the spread or the death counts. Florida reopened on September 25, 2020. While some forecasted disaster, the governor stood by his decision to remain open. Shortly thereafter, in late September, scientists from Harvard, Stanford, and Oxford Universities disavowed lockdowns. They declared them destructive and futile mitigation tactics.

The **unemployment numbers** have notably risen according to the National Bureau of Economic Research. Even the occasional stimulus check, as the federal government attempts to ease some of this financial hardship, it is not enough to pay the average family bills; even mortgage, food, electricity and water bill. All of these consequences must be considered for any future pandemics with recommendations for mitigation must include more than just virologists taking in account significant lockdowns may in fact be harmful.

As the world moves through the phases of **re-entry in our new normal lives**, whatever it will be, we are all fearful of changes and what a new life will be like. We keep our fears in check through our faith. We continue to know, deep down inside, that everything is going to be ok. We will get through this by hook or nail and get to a new normal at some point.

Throughout this pandemic, many have lost loved ones. Many have seen their **loved ones pass away** without their family nearby to keep the spread in check. At best they have seen them on their final day of life on a computer screen. Many have held private funerals because of no crowd rules, lacking the love and hugs of friends and family. They will never get that opportunity back.

Medical staffs have become the new heroes of our time. Nurses, doctors, and even maintenance staff who continued to report to the hospitals risked their own lives to help others. The true love of humanity showed its strength as these individuals showed through so strong. Then, one or more nurses, then one or more doctors, felt the stress rise to levels unbearable. They watched as more and more died and were taken from the facility in body bags. The strain became too great and they took their own lives. Their co-workers grieved, and cried, and were almost broken, but came back to the office and hospitals, taking every last bit of strength they had to help the sick. No one on this earth will forget those heroes and what they sacrificed to help their communities.

Those out of work stood in the **food bank lines**, hoping for a bit of more food as their funds began to run out. They needed to provide for their families and this was just one avenue to help in that need. They applied for unemployment benefits but spent weeks trying to just contact the unemployment offices as they were stretched to the limit responding to tens of thousands of new applications per day. They prayed for the day when their application was approved and hopefully could get an additional $600 per week during this pandemic. The United States stipend for families was set up and approved to help families get through the stay-at-home orders. Those within the general income guidelines

218

on their previous years' tax records would receive a check for $1200 per person and $500 for each child. This was intended to help pay mortgage or lease payments. Hopefully, with all the federal resources, families could get through this time.

Teachers and students have learned a **new way of learning**. Parents have learned a new appreciation for the teachers and the students have grown to appreciate their teachers in a new light. At home learning, or no learning, depending upon what the state dictated the public schools to do, have become the new norm, for now. It appears at this time, that most schools will remain closed for this school year and make arrangements to begin in the fall once again.

Colleges are continuing with online classes and plans to re-open in the fall. Of course, all of this depends upon the data at the time. Students, who were working jobs during the current school year, usually lost them and college students mostly went home. Most are looking for the fall to continue their education and get back into the swing of college life.

Singles and widows/widowers have become **lonelier than ever before** the COVID pandemic. While they may have had a full life prior to the virus, the stay-at-home orders have forced them to do just that…stay at home. There are no senior activities at the Senior Center; no walks on the beach; no bridge parties or shopping. They limit their grocery store trips and hopefully wear masks and gloves at any time outside of their own home. Family limits visitation to them and only checks on them from time to time to be sure they are ok and have what they need. The lack of touch and hugs has begun to take a toll on them as them become isolated. The older crowd is the high-risk group, prone to have severe symptoms if exposed, and more likely to die of the virus than other ages. So, they work in the yard if their old bones allow them, do crafts at home if they are crafty, paint another picture if they are an artsy, or write a book if they are a doodler. It does not ease the loneliness or fill the void of a hug but it gets them by. They miss their children and grandchildren, and even those interactions around the town. They will survive, if they do not contract it and wonder what they shall do or not do once all the stay-at-home orders are lifted.

The **small businessman and woman** wonder if they will still have a business when everything opens back up. Some even defy the orders and open up anyway. Some law enforcement officers cite the owners and others turn a blind eye. Others protest and beg the governors to open back up their states. Most owners are trying anything they can to maintain their businesses, inventory, leases, and most of all to help their employees. Federal grants are offered to owners which do not have to be paid back if they will use them to pay employees for the next few months. The funds do not seem to meet the demand and the operations of these funds seem shaky but are helping some. People try to order from take-out restaurants, but it is hard to compete with chain hardware stores for the dollars which are becoming scare. We shall see what happens in the next few months.

Families are hurting. The stress of the lock-downs has created closeness in many instances with family members staying in close contact via telephone and video chats while others seem worlds apart, unable to see each other at all. Husbands are getting on the nerves of their wives and vice versa. Staying together 24 hours per day is not the vacation it started out to be months ago. These challenges are causing some to grow and others to crumble. It has become a challenge for many and a blessing for others.

While the United States seems to be recovering from this pandemic, other countries like India remain on high alert facing increased cases and deaths from Covid. By May 1, 2021, reports indicate many large towns are short of oxygen to help the ill and large numbers are dying. This week their death toll topped 211,000 but some say it may be ten times higher than the reported numbers. Morgues and funeral homes are so full that bodies are being cremated in parking lots in New Delhi. This second wave of Covid has hit India extremely hard. India has currently reported over 19 million cases. Numbers continue to rise. Brazil also continued to fight Covid deaths which were now passing 400,000. Vaccinations continue across the globe. It is not over yet. The mutation B.617 variant is the culpable virus causing such death in India. The U. S. and other countries are gathering aid to help providing oxygen as thousands die daily.

In the U. S. on May of 2021, President Joe Biden announced that we can now go outside without masks and attend ballgames without a mask, if we have had a vaccination, of course. As of this date, estimates are that about half of Americans eligible for vaccines are vaccinated. The whole issue of being outdoors, and even wearing a mask at all outdoors for the past year, seemed illogical to many. One high school track runner recently lost consciousness at the finish line due to lack of oxygen because of the required mask. That coach is now working to get that requirement changed to protect the young athletes. Sometimes pure common sense needs to rule. Some just shake their heads wondering how the leaders of our country can make such demands of the common citizen. How much power does the government actually have over a person? The feds exerted a lot of power and *guidelines* during this past year, extending far beyond what we might have ever imaged two years ago. We hope this passes and the pandemic becomes a nightmare of a memory; never forgotten but left in the past. We look forward to taking back the rights to make our own decisions regarding our jobs, health and lives.

Regardless of the state of things as of this date, the **selflessness continues to show** itself as we see flags fly high. The Spirit of Americanism and country support has grown strong. The strength of certain individuals and leaders had brought us together as one; or most of those I know. We each face our own challenges and we continue to get up and face the day. We continue to look for the new normal and watch daily updates on the news. We continue to love on our animals, call those we cherish, and wonder what the future will hold. May God bless us all throughout this world and restore us to a fully functioning society; better and stronger than before.

Former **President George W. Bush**, posted a video chat on May 2, 2020, sharing his thoughts on the virus and impact on everyone. His words hold true today in

2021. He said, "This is a challenging and solemn time in the life of our nation and world. A remorseless invisible enemy threatens the elderly and vulnerable among us. A disease that can quickly take breathe and life. Medical professionals are risking their own health for the health of others and we are deeply grateful."

"Officials at every level are setting out the **requirements of public health** that protect us all. And we all need to do our part. The disease also threatens broader damage; harm to our sense of safety, security, and community. The larger challenge we share is to confront an outbreak of fear and loneliness. And it is frustrating that all of the normal tools of compassion, a hug or a touch can bring the opposite of the good that we intend. In this case we serve our neighbor by separating from them. We cannot allow physical separation to become emotional isolation. This requires us to be not only compassionate but creative in our outreach. And people across the nation are using the tools of technology in the cause of solidarity," he said.

President Bush continued with, "In this time of testing, we need to remember a few things. First, let us remember we have faced times of testing before. Following 9-11, I saw a great nation rise as one to honor the brave, to grieve with the grieving, and to embrace unavoidable new duties. And I have no doubt, none at all, that the spirit of service and sacrifice is alive and well in America.

He said, "Second, let us remember that empathy and simple kindness are essential and powerful tools of national recovery. Even at an appropriate social distance, we can find ways to be present in the lives of others to ease their anxiety and share their burdens. Third, let's remember that the suffering we experience as a nation does not fall evenly."

He continued with, "In the days that come, it will be especially important to care in practical ways for the elderly, the ill and the unemployed. Finally, let us remember how small our differences are in the face of this shared threat. In the final analysis, we are not partisan combatants; we are human beings equally vulnerable and equally wonderful in the site of God. We rise or fall together and we are determined to rise. God Bless you all."

In addition, financial hardships, suicides, and a host of additional mental, physical and emotional problems have come into the spotlight as a result of quarantine, sickness, death, unemployment, and other affects of COVID-19 on our country, states, communities, families and individuals. Every person has dealt with the virus in their own manner; some in a positive manner and others in negative ways. Each individual reading this text is encouraged to document their own personal story in the blank pages forthcoming. And in so doing, work toward the potential to internalize and recognize how this virus has affected him or her. What is known and readily accepted is that this virus has changed us all in one way or another. Children will remember the year they were not in school. Workers will remember how their jobs just disappeared at the stroke of a pen by their own governors. Children grieved their parents in nursing homes being unable to visit, touch and hold.

Families barely fathomed how it would be burying their dead with no one allowed to attend the funeral.

Political situations evolved amid elections and also various races and police. The entire community balances of law and order were turned upside down with riots and crowds burning buildings, setting up law free zones, attacking government buildings, tearing down statutes, and pretty much doing whatever the crowd wanted to do in certain towns and cities. Other cities just watched this madness on television or read accounts on the computer and in newspapers. Even an attempted takeover of the Capitol Building in Washington, DC occurred with people overrunning the building while Congress was in session forcing senators and representatives to escape via protected hallways and exits. The entire world watched as order was eventually restored and Congress came back into session later that evening to document the results of the recent Presidential election, establishing the election of President Joe Biden.

Faith without Fear

While it is unclear who is sponsoring the signs, they have been spotted throughout the county, state and nation...*Faith without Fear*. These small yard signs describe perfectly in such a few words what the majority of people of faith feel about this pandemic. However, many consider the implication that the end of this world may be coming to an end. The Bible references so many verses which talk of the plagues and destruction of this world as we know it. It occurs primarily in the Old Testament.

"The Bible describes numerous occasions when God brought plagues and diseases on His people and on His enemies "To make you see my power" (Exodus 9:14, 16). He used plagues on Egypt to force Pharaoh to free the Israelites from bondage, while sparing His people from being affected by them (Exodus 12:13; 15:26), thus indicating His sovereign control over diseases and other afflictions."[82]

Beyond the verses of being stricken with disease, our Lord also promised to heal his children.

2 Chronicles 7:14 - If my people, which are called by my name, shall humble themselves, and pray, and seek my face, and turn from their wicked ways; then will I hear from heaven, and will forgive their sin, and will heal their land.

In the King James Bible, He told us not to fear:

Isaiah 41:10 - Fear thou not; for I [am] with thee: be not dismayed; for I [am] thy God: I will strengthen thee; yea, I will help thee; yea, I will uphold thee with the right hand of my righteousness.

---

[82] Got Questions? Your answers. https://www.gotquestions.org/pandemic-diseases.html.

2 Timothy 1:7 - For God hath not given us the spirit of fear; but of power, and of love, and of a sound mind.

Psalms 34:4 - I sought the LORD, and he heard me, and delivered me from all my fears.

Proverbs 29:25 - The fear of man bringeth a snare: but whoso putteth his trust in the LORD shall be safe.

Philippians 4:6 - Be careful for nothing; but in everything by prayer and supplication with thanksgiving let your requests be made known unto God.

In the meantime, most churches were closed with services only available for viewing on the computer. Some which have opened for large congregations have met the wrath of the law enforcement and city leaders; chastised for unhealthy environments which spread the virus. One must wonder how many people are watching and feeling the faith while not being among his children in the church building. By May of 2021, churches began to open and hold regular services with spacing in the pews and suggesting but not requiring masks. It seemed to be working well as services got back to the new normal of 2021.

Our **world had changed**. Every situation changed us. We would never be the same person as before Covid. Just when we thought sports might return to fans being allowed to attend, in June of 2021, at the Jack Nicklaus PGA tournament, the unthinkable happened to the leading player. In Dublin Ohio, the game on June 5, 2021, changed at the 18th green at Muirfield Village. While Jon Rahm one of the top golfers in the world took a brief rain break at the 18th hole, PGA Tour officials surround Rahm and explain he must withdraw from the tournament after testing positive for COVID-19. He was in a sic-stroke lead and had just tied the 54-hole scoring record at the memorial.

Rahm was one of the contract tracing individuals who was noted to have been near a person who also tested positive. Under the games rules, he would have to test after each round and following the completion of a weather-delayed second round when he tested positive.

Rahm had been involved in contract tracing after being in close proximity with a person who had COVID-19. Under the circuit's protocols he was allowed to remain in the tournament but he had to test after each round and following the completion of the weather-delayed second round he tested positive. Viewers and fan on scene were flabbergasted just shaking their heads in disbelief. A champion was disqualified on the last hole.

But we remained hopeful, had faith in our God, and knew that a better day was coming. The battle to regain normalcy, whatever that is to each individual, had not been won yet. It will come.

Adversity came to our lives and we faced it dead on. We met the challenge. The young, old, weary, wealthy, poor, and all in between, stood together to keep moving forward. We tended to our sick, we buried our dead, and we embraced our loved ones when we all needed it most. Whether we walked it alone, or banded together with friends and family, we learned; we suffered; and we loved. Tomorrow came and we forged ahead to an uncertain future. Only time will tell what the long-term impacts of this disease will be world-wide, country-wide, state-wide, county-wide; or within the family or individual. The next chapter remains unwritten. It is for you, to write your own story of how this pandemic turns out and this author encourages you to do so for future generations to read.

It is time to go back to enjoying our normal activities. Back to work. Back to school. Back to church. Back to family reunions. And back to going out to eat and shopping. Back to travel and perhaps some type of normal life.   Globally. We have not reached that point yet, but know it will be coming. Hopefully, soon.

We saw and felt many things during this deadly pandemic. We still had *Hope, Faith and Love*. May God put his arms around you, dear reader. May God bless you, my friend. And may you walk in his light; forever protected by angel wings, with **Faith over Fear**.

Mark 9:23 –

And Jesus said to him, "If you can believe, all things are possible.

June 8, 2021

Chapter 10

My Story of the Pandemic

Name:

_____

Address: _____

City/Town/Zip:
_____

Family members living with me:

_____
_____
_____
_____

Where I was, Who was important in my life, what our daily routine became, who I know got ill, who I know died, how I felt at the beginning and throughout the pandemic, what lessons I learned while going through this experience, what I wish my children and grandchildren could learn from my experience, and how this experience has made me into a stronger, more caring person, or what anxieties I felt during this time. Was I lonely? What I happy? What bothered me? What did I do to help others? Who was so caring and helped me during this experience? What do I look forward to doing in the future? Who do I look forward to seeing? What am I grateful for? My prayer for my family….

My Story:

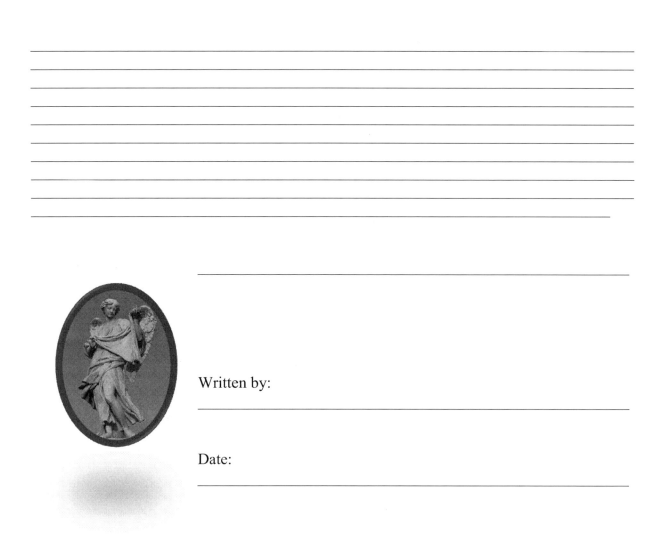

Written by:

_____

Date:

_____

PS. Remember to continue writing even after you fill up this book. Just let your loved ones know that you have a journal.

2 Timothy 4:7 –

I have fought the good fight, I have finished the race, I have kept the faith.

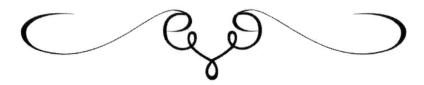

Appendix

North Carolina and Brunswick County

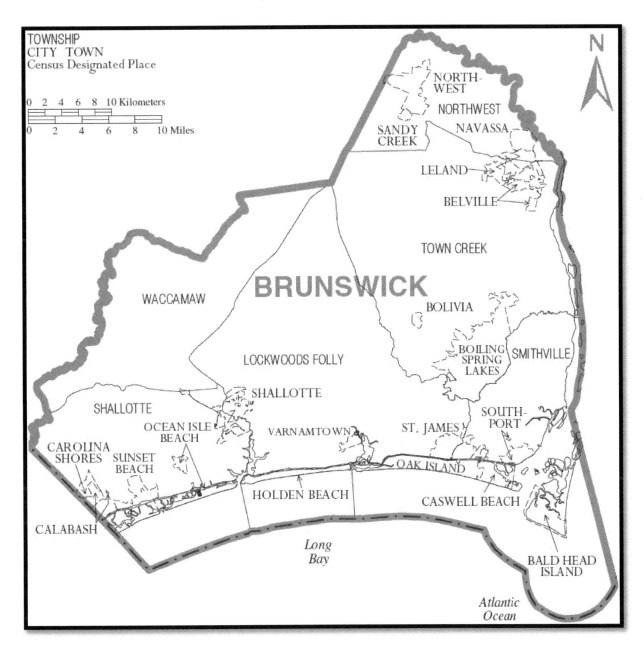

Brunswick County, North Carolina may be a good rural community to examine for the progression of the COVID-19 virus experience both in North Carolina and across the nation. Brunswick County, located in southeastern North Carolina and bordered by the Atlantic Ocean is a vacation destination for many. With a growing permanent population and a large percentage of senior citizens over the age of 65, Brunswick County officials faced the challenge of healthy practices following Governors Roy Coopers' guidelines. Here is how the situation appeared in mid April of 2020.

North Carolina COVID-19 Positive Case Statistics on April 15, 2020

North Carolina: 5,123 known cases

                    431 currently hospitalized

                    117 deaths

Of these cases, 44% of the cases are male and 53% are female. Two percent are unknown. 69% of the deaths are male and 30 percent female.

Age-wise, the cases breakdown as follows:

Age Group	Percent of Cases	Percent of Deaths
0-17	1%	0%
18-24	7%	0%
25-49	38%	7%
50-64	28%	12%
65+	25%	79%

Guidance from the NC Department of Health and Human Services to the Public: (March 23, 2020)

•Stay home and call your doctor, if needed.

•Stay home even if you have fever, cough without shortness of breath or difficulty breathing. However, call the doctor if you need medical care.

•If you are at a higher risk, and have symptoms of fever or cough, be sure to call your doctor. Those of higher risk are considered: 65 years of age or older, living in a nursing home or long-term care facility, or have a high-risk health condition. Some of those might include chronic lung disease, asthma, heart disease, compromised immune system, severe obesity, body mass index of 40 or higher, or other underlying medical conditions such as diabetes, renal failure or liver disease.

•Call your doctor if you have: shortness of breath, chest pain or pressure, blue lips, difficulty breathing or confusion. (It seems to this author (and others) that if you are at the point of blue lips, there is a real emergency!)

According to the NCDHHS, most people do not need a test. Reason: because you may expose yourself to others who have it if you do not, and if you have it, you may give it to others. (Not sure I understand this logic.)

They also explain that there is no treatment for COVID-19. For people with mild symptoms who don't need medical care, getting a test will not change what you or our doctor does.

•Isolate Yourself. Stay home and separate yourself from other people in the home as much as possible.

•Maintain social distancing policies. This is touted as the best policy to ensure our health system has sufficient capacity to manage the growing number of COVID-19 infections. Social distancing involves us staying at least six feet away from any other person no matter where we are when away from home.

As noted, many experts were fearful of the number of cases requiring hospitalization and overtaxing the staff, beds and equipment needed for severe cases, particularly the ventilators.

April 25-26: Six more symptoms have been added to the positive COVID-19 diagnosis: (in addition to the cough, fever and shortness of breath.)

   --Chills

   --Repeated shaking

   --Muscle pain

   --Sore throat

   --Loss of sense of smell and taste

North Carolina Statistics on April 27, 2020

In North Carolina, similarly to the past 40 days, 60% of the deaths are male and 39% female. Males have been documented as 48% of the cases and females with 51% of the positive cases with 2% unknown. In North Carolina there have been over 9,142 cases diagnosed with 306 deaths. 86% of the number of deaths in North Carolina are in the age group of over 65; however, of the percent of cases diagnosed, only 24% are those in that age category.

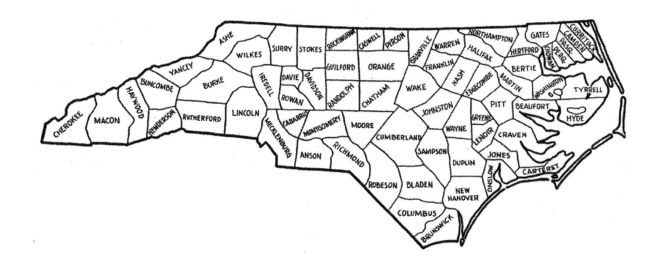

83

North Carolina [84]

May 6 and one week later, May 11th, 2020.

Date	May 6	May 11
Cases	12,758	15,045
Deaths		550
Hospitalized	477	464
# counties	99	99
Tested	164,482	195,865

---

[83] Map courtesy of https://www.fotolip.com/north-carolina-county-map-5568.html

[84] North Carolina Department of Health and Human Services. https://COVID19.ncdhhs.gov/dashboard#by-race-ethnicity .

Of these cases,   3% were 0 to 17 years of age

          8% were 18 to 24

      42% were 25 to 49   3% of deaths

      25% were 50 to 64   11% of death

      21% were aged 65 or older   86% of deaths

Additional criteria noted included:

Race	May 11 Cases	May 11 % of Cases	May 11 COVID Deaths	May 11 % of COVID Deaths
American Indian; Alaska Native	105	1	1	0
Asian	277	3	6	1
Black or African American	3,841	35	179	34
Native Hawaiian or Pacific Islander	22	0	1	0
White	5,840	53	314	60
Other	915	8	20	4
Ethnicity				
Hispanic	2,526	26	20	4
Non-Hispanic	7,365	74	442	96

Cases by Gender	May 11 Cases	May 11 Deaths
Male	48%	53%
Female	51%	47%

Race data is missing for 4,045 laboratory-confirmed cases and 29 deaths.

2 Ethnicity data are missing for 5,154 laboratory-confirmed cases and 88 deaths.

All data are preliminary and may change as cases are investigated.

3Gender may be unknown and account for less than 100% reported.

2020 Statistics across North Carolina by County

County	May 6 Cases	May 6 Deaths	May 11 Cases	May 11 Deaths
Alamance	128	3	178	5
Alexander	6	0	12	0
Alleghany	7	0	8	0
Anson	31	0	38	0
Ashe	5	0	10	0
Beaufort	21	0	25	0
Bertie	53	2	61	2
Bladen	40	1	54	1
Brunswick	49	2	50	2

Buncombe	78	4	101	4
Burke	117	10	137	11
Cabarrus	323	16	350	17
Caldwell	43	0	60	0
Camden	2	0	2	0
Carteret	28	3	31	3
Caswell	36	0	41	1
Catawba	63	1	82	2
Chatham	412	11	458	11
Cherokee	19	1	18	1
Chowan	7	0	11	0
Clay	5	0	5	0
Cleveland	48	2	50	2
Columbus	175	11	205	14
Craven	43	4	55	4
Cumberland	318	8	351	9
Currituck	5	0	9	0
Dare	14	1	17	1
Davidson	186	9	205	10
Davie	31	2	36	2
Duplin	146	3	258	3
Durham	793	27	873	32
Edgecombe	128	5	155	7
Forsythe	308	5	379	5
Franklin	106	20	111	20
Gaston	155	4	175	5
Gates	10	0	11	0

Graham	2	0	2	0
Granville	161	5	167	6
Greene	22	0	36	1
Guilford	507	35	609	38
Halifax	73	1	94	1
Harnett	192	10	228	13
Haywood	15	0	17	0
Henderson	213	22	227	28
Hertford	46	1	51	1
Hoke	103	0	123	0
Hyde	1	0	1	0
Iredell	136	5	153	5
Jackson	20	1	21	1
Johnston	188	16	209	16
Jones	19	2	20	2
Lee	207	1	227	1
Lenoir	91	4	122	4
Lincoln	37	0	39	0
Macon	3	1	3	1
Madison	1	0	1	0
Martin	25	1	31	1
McDowell	28	1	29	1
Mecklenburg	1,850	57	2,134	62
Mitchell	5	0	5	6
Montgomery	41	2	42	2
Moore	106	3	111	9
Nash	104	3	121	3

New Hanover	84	3	97	3
Northampton	93	4	106	7
Onslow	52	2	54	2
Orange	230	20	253	33
Pamlico	8	0	8	0
Pasquotank	38	2	81	3
Pender	19	1	39	1
Perquimans	14	2	17	2
Person	23	1	31	1
Pitt	145	2	169	22
Polk	27	0	29	0
Randolph	275	4	354	6
Richmond	65	2	94	2
Robeson	288	3	391	44
Rockingham	34	2	42	2
Rowan	439	24	488	24
Rutherford	145	5	154	5
Sampson	108	1	167	1
Scotland	32	0	41	0
Stanley	30	4	29	4
Stokes	10	0	11	0
Surry	20	1	43	1
Swain	4	0	5	0
Transylvania	7	0	7	0
Tyrrell	4	0	4	0
Union	275	13	301	16
Vance	120	10	162	12

Wake	937	21	1,048	23
Warren	18	0	23	0
Washington	25	3	25	3
Watauga	8	0	9	0
Wayne	687	12	752	13
Wilkes	147	1	242	1
Wilson	184	7	214	8
Yadkin	27	1	54	1
Yancy	1	0	9	0

All data are preliminary and may change as cases are investigated.

North Carolina Map Chart on next page is dated May 11, 2020. It demonstrates the rise and decline of cases, over time, in our state from March 3 to May 11.

Brunswick County, North Carolina

Statistics on April 15, 2020, show that in Brunswick County, North Carolina, 42 people[85], which includes those who came here from other states and are classified as non-residents have COVID-19. Those non-residents are actually counted in their home states, but came here and brought the virus with them. Eight Corona victims in our state have died.[86] This in itself makes many local residents angry when our count is relatively low in comparison to many other locations around our country. As of this date, the current statistics are shown below and shared by the Brunswick County Emergency Management Office to keep all of the primary businesses and groups aware of what is happening in this county.

COVID-19 Partner Briefing: Operational Day 34: April 15, 2020

---

[85] April 16, 2020. Brunswick County, NC COVID-19 Daily Briefing.
[86] IBID.

Brunswick County Health and Human Services

Case Count

2,034,425 cases globally (133,261 deaths)

619,607 cases in the United States (27,760 deaths)

5,123 cases in North Carolina (117 deaths)

35 Cases in Brunswick County (1 death)[87]

Number of test samples in the county - 960

Pending Test Sample Results – 28

Positive Test Results reported to the county – 35

Negative Test Results reported to the county – 897.

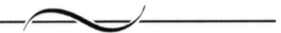

Brunswick County Resident COVID-19 Positive Case Statistics

Gender: 49% are male and 51% are female.

Age	Percent of Cases	Percent of Deaths
0-17	0%	0%
18-24	6%	0%
25-49	14%	0%
50-64	43%	0%
65+	37%	100%

Of the 35 (note which does not include nonresidents in our county) 4 are isolated at home, 1 isolated in the hospital, 1 death and 29 currently recovered.

Of the 8 nonresidents COVID-19 cases as of this date:

---

[87] Count does not include 8 nonresident Cases and 1 death in our county of a nonresident. Numbers current as of 4/15/2020 4 pm John Hopkins Data.

0 isolated at home, 2 isolated at the hospital, 1 death, 4 currently recovered, and 2 transferred monitoring to home residence. The one death was over the age of 65 with others totally 71% of the nonresident COVID-19 cases over the age of 65. The other cases were designated as between the ages of 25 and 49 at 29 % of the cases.

These test results have been reported daily for the past 34 days and bring up many more questions than they seem to answer. While results throughout the United States vary from less than one thousand per state to over 7,000 dying each day (New York).

*Why are the results divided into resident and nonresident when they were detected and treated in our county? Even more, why were they allowed to leave highly infected locations such as New York to come to our county? Of course, we realize that these folks are ill and perhaps wanted to see the ocean once again, visit their vacation homes one more time, or generally so frightened by the place where they reside that they decided to come here to escape the virus; bringing it with them.

*Where are the primary cases located within our county? Are they in the Northern section (Leland areas), the Southern section (Southport area) or the Western section (Shallotte area)? Are we better off knowing or not? Health officials have decided we shall not know but word travels and we know that one of those transplants ended up in the Holden Beach area and one in the Southport area. We can only guess the remainder. Later the zip code area will be known and they seem to be all over, generally.

Why were so many of the tests coming back negative? Is there a defect in the test itself? Perhaps only those who are reported to have traveled out of country or been exposed to a now diagnosed case or those who have extreme symptoms requiring hospitalization tested?

Why is it so difficult for those who have mild to moderate symptoms to get tested? They started out testing folks for the flu first and then if they failed the flu test, were given the Corona test. But that soon turned into unless you needed hospitalization or known exposure, sorry no test. That happened to my daughter.

We wonder if there are still drive through areas for testing and what the requirements are to get a test if you are not having respiratory symptoms or in close contact with someone who has it. We wonder if testing is possible for those with symptoms such as low fever, nausea, extreme tiredness and headache.

A retired virologist residing here in the Holden Beach area, Dr. John McEntire, stated, "I believe they are only testing very advanced cases so that results are essentially meaningless. If we don't test someone then we don't have a sick person to deal with. The number of infected is probably much higher. Interestingly, that also pushes up the fatality rate. These tests are readily available now, and run mostly on existing platforms already available in hospital and clinic labs. Why wouldn't they do this?"

The Brunswick County Health Services are recommending the following factions as of April 15, 2020.

Incident Objectives

    Continue to monitor virus spread.

    Make decisions and any recommendations based on data received in the Emergency Operations Center.

    Continue to develop surge plan protocols.

    Congregate Care Intervention Task Force is Operational.

Brunswick County COVID-19 Partner Briefing Operational Day 46

April 27, 2020

As for the past 46 days, the Brunswick County, North Carolina Emergency Management Office, led by Ed Cornrow, and the Brunswick County Health Services Office, led by David Stanley, have coordinated a written briefing distributed to all partners, agencies, schools, law enforcement, hospitals, utilities, fire, rescue, etc. and is available online for all citizens, updating the current situation daily.

As of April 27th, Brunswick County recorded 43 cases with two deaths. They also recorded ten more cases with two deaths of nonresidents. These statistics are broken down into daily statistics by gender and age for positive results and deaths. There are only 17 tests pending results.

May 3, 2020

    On May the 3rd, some airlines announced that all flyers will be required to wear masks while on the plane. They will also be required to wear masks when checking in and on the premises inside the buildings to protect employees.

    In Oklahoma, a requirement for face masks for customers in stores, led to physical confrontations with employees in the stores. After that sporadic outbreak, the governor walked that requirement back but still requires employees to wear masks. Other states watch as other states slowly open.

    On May 5, 2020, Governor Roy Cooper of North Carolina provided a new executive order. Phase One has begun:

State of Carolina

ROY COOPER, GOVERNOR

May 05, 2020

EXECUTIVE ORDER NO. 138[88]

EASING RESTRICTIONS ON TRAVEL, BUSINESS OPERATIONS, AND MASS GATHERINGS: PHASE 1

WHEREAS, on March 10, 2020, the undersigned issued Executive Order No. 1 16 which declared a State of Emergency to coordinate the State's response and protective actions to address the Coronavirus Disease 2019 ("COVID- 19") public health emergency and provide for the health, safety, and welfare of residents and visitors located in North Carolina; and

WHEREAS, on March 11, 2020, the World Health Organization declared COVID-19 a global pandemic; and

WHEREAS, on March 13, 2020, the President of the United States issued an emergency declaration for all states, tribes, territories, and the District of Columbia, retroactive to March 1, 2020, and the President declared that the COVID-19 pandemic in the United States constitutes a national emergency; and

WHEREAS, on March 25, 2020, the President approved a Major Disaster Declaration, FEMA-4487-DR, for the State of North Carolina; and

WHEREAS, in responding to the COVID-19 pandemic, and for the purpose of protecting the health, safety, and welfare of the people of North Carolina, the undersigned has issued Executive Order Nos. 116-122, 124-125, 129-131, and 133-136; and

WHEREAS, more than ten thousand people in North Carolina have had laboratory confirmed cases of COVID-19, and hundreds of people in North Carolina have died from the disease; and

WHEREAS, hospital administrators and health care providers have expressed concerns that unless the spread of COVID-19 is limited, existing health care facilities may be insufficient to care for those who become sick; and

WHEREAS, the undersigned and the Secretary of Health and Human Services have directed hospitals, physicians' practices, and other health care entities to undertake significant actions as part of North Carolina's emergency response to address the COVID-19 pandemic; and

WHEREAS, slowing and controlling community spread of COVID-19 is critical to ensuring that the state's healthcare facilities remain able to accommodate those who require medical assistance; and

---

[88] NC Executive Order 138. Phase One of the opening of North Carolina. May 5, 2020.

WHEREAS, the continued community spread of COVID-19 within North Carolina requires the state to continue some measures to slow the spread of this virus during the pandemic; and

WHEREAS, since the issuance of executive orders to slow the spread of COVID-19, North Carolina has "flattened the curve" and prevented a surge or spike in cases across the state, and North Carolina has also increased its capacity for testing, tracing and the availability of personal protective equipment ("PPE"); and

WHEREAS, despite the overall stability in key metrics, North Carolina's daily case counts of COVID-19 continue to increase slightly in the context of increased testing, demonstrating the state must remain vigilant in its work to slow the spread of the virus; and

WHEREAS, the risk of COVID-19 transmission remains high, particularly with regard to indoor settings with an increased likelihood of close contact; and

WHEREAS, people in North Carolina are encouraged to use a cloth face covering to reduce the spread of COVID-19, but some populations may experience increased anxiety and fear of bias and being profiled if wearing face coverings in public spaces; and

WHEREAS, if someone is the target of ethnic or racial intimidation as the result of adhering to the mask provision or as a result of the pandemic, they are encouraged to report the matter to law enforcement or another government entity; and

WHEREAS, Executive Order No. 116 invoked the Emergency Management Act, and authorizes the undersigned to exercise the powers and duties set forth therein to direct and aid in the response to, recovery from, and mitigation against emergencies; and

WHEREAS, pursuant to N.C. Gen. Stat. 166A-19.10(b)(2), the undersigned may make, amend, or rescind necessary orders, rules, and regulations within the limits of the authority conferred upon the Governor in the Emergency Management Act; and

WHEREAS, N.C. Gen. Stat. 166A-19. authorizes and empowers the undersigned to delegate Gubernatorial vested authority under the Emergency Management Act and to provide for the sub-delegation of that authority; and

WHEREAS, N.C. Gen. Stat.   gives the undersigned the authority to "cooperate and coordinate" with the President of the United States; and

WHEREAS, pursuant to N.C. Gen. Stat. 166A-19.12(3)(e), the Division of Emergency Management must coordinate with the State Health Director to revise the North Carolina Emergency Operations Plan as conditions change, including making revisions to set "the appropriate conditions for quarantine and isolation in order to prevent the further transmission of disease," and following this coordination, the Emergency Management Director and the State Health Director have recommended that the Governor develop and order the plan and actions identified in this Executive Order; and

WHEREAS, pursuant to N.C. Gen. Stat. S 166A-19.23 in conjunction with N.C. Gen. Stat. 75-37 and 75-38, the undersigned may issue a declaration that shall trigger the prohibitions against excessive pricing during states of disaster, states of emergency or abnormal market disruptions; and

WHEREAS, pursuant to N.C. Gen. Stat. 166A-19.30(a)(l), the undersigned may utilize all available state resources as reasonably necessary to cope with an emergency, including the transfer and direction of personnel or functions of state agencies or units thereof for the purpose of performing or facilitating emergency services; and

WHEREAS, pursuant to N.C. Gen. Stat. 166A-19.30(a)(2), the undersigned may take such action and give such directions to state and local law enforcement officers and agencies as may be reasonable and necessary for the purpose of securing compliance with the provisions of the Emergency Management Act and with the orders, rules, and regulations made there under; and

WHEREAS, pursuant to N.C. Gen. Stat. the undersigned has determined that local control of the emergency is insufficient to assure adequate protection for lives and property of North Carolinians because not all local authorities have enacted such appropriate ordinances or issued such appropriate declarations restricting the operation of businesses and limiting person-to-person contact, thus needed control cannot be imposed locally; and

WHEREAS, pursuant to N.C. Gen. Stat. 166A-19.30(c)(ii), the undersigned has determined that local control of the emergency is insufficient to assure adequate protection for lives and property of North Carolinians because some but not all local authorities have taken implementing steps under such ordinances or declarations, if enacted or declared, in order to effectuate control over the emergency that has arisen; and

WHEREAS, pursuant to N.C. Gen. Stat. the undersigned has determined that local control of the emergency is insufficient to assure adequate protection for lives and property of North Carolinians because the area in which the emergency exists spreads across local jurisdictional boundaries and the legal control measures of the jurisdictions are conflicting or uncoordinated to the extent that efforts to protect life and property are, or unquestionably will be, severely hampered; and

WHEREAS, pursuant to N.C. Gen. Stat. the undersigned has determined that local control of the emergency is insufficient to assure adequate protection of lives and property of North Carolinians because the scale of the emergency is so great that it exceeds the capability of local authorities to cope with it; and

WHEREAS, N.C. Gen. Stat. 166A-19.30(c) in conjunction with N.C. Gen. Stat. 166A19.31 (b)(l) authorizes the undersigned to prohibit and restrict the movement of people in public places; and

WHEREAS, N.C. Gen. Stat. 166A-19.30(c) in conjunction with N.C. Gen. Stat. 166A authorizes the undersigned to prohibit and restrict the operation of offices, business establishments, and other places to and from which people may travel or at which they may congregate; and

WHEREAS, N.C. Gen. Stat. 166A-19.30(c) in conjunction with N.C. Gen. Stat. S 166A authorizes the undersigned to prohibit and restrict other activities or conditions, the control of which may be reasonably necessary to maintain order and protect lives or property during a state of emergency; and

WHEREAS, pursuant to N.C. Gen. Stat. when the undersigned imposes the prohibitions and restrictions enumerated in N.C. Gen. Stat. 166A-19.31(b), the undersigned may amend or rescind the prohibitions and restrictions imposed by local authorities; and

WHEREAS, pursuant to N.C. Gen. Stat. during a Gubernatorial declared State of Emergency, the undersigned has the power to "give such directions to State and local law enforcement officers and agencies as may be reasonable and necessary for the purpose of securing compliance with the provisions of this Article."

NOW, THEREFORE, by the authority vested in me as Governor by the Constitution and the laws of the State ofN0flh Carolina, IT IS ORDERED:

Section 1. Definitions.

In this Executive Order:

l. "Allowable Activities" are defined in Section 2(C) of this Executive Order.

2. "Bars" means establishments that are not eating establishments or restaurants as defined in N.C. Gen. Stat. 18B-1000(2) and 18B-1000(6) and have a permit to sell alcoholic beverages for onsite consumption under N.C. Gen. Stat. 18B-1001.

3. "Face Covering" means a covering of the nose and mouth by wearing a cloth covering or mask for the purpose of ensuring the physical health or safety of the wearer or others as defined in Session Law 2020-3 s. 4.3(a). In the context of the COVID-19 emergency, the Face Covering predominantly functions to protect other people more than the wearer.

4. "Home" means someone's house, place of residence, or current place of abode.

5. "Mass Gathering" is defined in Section 6(A) of this Executive Order.

6. "Recommendations to Promote Social Distancing and Reduce Transmission" are defined in Section 2(A) of this Executive Order.

7. "Restaurants" means permitted food establishments, under N.C. Gen. Stat. 130A-248, and other establishments that both prepare and serve food. This includes, but is not limited to, restaurants, cafeterias, food halls, dining halls, food courts, and food kiosks. This includes not only free-standing locations but also locations within other businesses or facilities, including, but not limited to airports, shopping centers, educational institutions, or private or members-only clubs where food and beverages are permitted to be consumed on premises.

8. "Retail Business" means any business in which customers enter a space to purchase goods or services, including but not limited to grocery stores, convenience stores, large-format retail stores, pharmacies, banks, ABC stores, hardware stores, and vehicle dealerships. "Retail Business" also includes retail establishments operated by the State, its political subdivisions, or agencies thereof.

Section 2.   Allowable Activities for Individuals Outside the Home.

All individuals currently in the State of North Carolina may undertake Allowable Activities permitted by this Executive Order. Otherwise, individuals are ordered to stay at home.

A.   Recommendations to Promote Social Distancing and Reduce Transmission. Individuals leaving their residence for Allowable Activities are strongly advised to take the following steps to reduce transmission:

1. Maintain at least six (6) feet social distancing from other individuals, with the exception of family or household members.

2. Wear a cloth Face Covering when leaving home and wear it inside all public settings such as grocery stores, pharmacies, or other retail or public-serving businesses. A Face Covering should also be worn outdoors when you cannot maintain at least six (6) feet distancing from other people with the exception of family or household members. These coverings function to protect other people more than the wearer.

3.   Carry hand sanitizer with you when leaving home, and use it frequently.

4. Wash hands using soap and water for at least twenty (20) seconds as frequently as possible.

5.   Regularly clean high-touch surfaces such as steering wheels, wallets, phones.

6.   Stay at home if sick.

B. High-Risk Individuals: People who are at high risk of severe illness from COVID-19 continue to be strongly encouraged to stay home and travel only for absolutely essential purposes. The Centers for Disease Control and Prevention ("CDC") defines high-risk individuals as people 65 years or older, and people of any age who have serious underlying medical conditions including people who are immune-compromised, or with chronic lung disease, moderate-to-severe asthma, serious heart conditions, severe obesity, diabetes, with chronic kidney disease undergoing dialysis, or liver disease.

C. Allowable Activities: People may leave their residence for the following Allowable Activities. When engaged in activities outside their home, individuals should, as much as reasonably possible, adhere to the Recommendations to Promote Social Distancing and Reduce Transmission above, and are subject to any applicable Mass Gathering or activity restrictions pursuant to Sections 3 to 7 of this Executive Order.

1.   For health and safety. People may leave their homes to engage in activities or perform tasks for the health and safety of themselves, their family or household members, or those

who are unable to or should not leave their home (including, but not limited to, pets). For example, and without limitation, people may leave their homes to seek emergency services, obtain medical supplies or medication, or visit a health care professional or veterinarian.

2. To look for and obtain goods and services. People may leave their homes to look for or obtain goods and services from a business or operation that is not closed by a current Executive Order. This authorization does not include attendance as a spectator at a sporting event, concert, or other performance.

3. To engage in outdoor activity. People may leave their homes to engage in outdoor activities unless prohibited by this Executive Order.

4. For work. People may leave their homes to perform work at any business, nonprofit, government, or other organization that is not closed by this Executive Order. For example, and without limitation, people can leave the house for employment, or to serve as a contractor at a for-profit business, a nonprofit organization, a part of government, a single person business, a sole proprietorship, or any other kind of entity or operation.

5. To look for work. People may leave their homes to seek employment.

6. To take care of others. People may leave their homes to care for or assist a family member, friend, or pet in another household, and to transport family members, friends, or pets as allowed by this Executive Order. This includes attending weddings and funerals.

7. To worship or exercise First Amendment rights. People may leave their homes to travel to and from a place of worship or exercise any other rights protected under the First Amendment to the U.S. Constitution and its North Carolina counterparts.

8. To travel between places of residence. People may leave their homes to return to or to travel between one's place or places of residence. This includes, but is not limited to, child custody or visitation arrangements.

9. To volunteer. People may leave their homes to volunteer with organizations that provide charitable and social services.

10. To attend small outdoor get-togethers. People may travel to another person's home for social purposes, so long as no more than ten (10) people gather and the activity occurs outside.

11. To provide or receive government services. People may leave their homes for governmental services. Nothing in this Executive Order shall prohibit anyone from performing actions for, or receiving services from, the state or any of its political subdivisions, boards, commissions, or agencies. This Executive Order does not apply to the United States government.

D.   Specific Situations.

l. Homelessness. Individuals experiencing homelessness are exempt from the order to stay at home, but they are strongly urged to obtain shelter and services that allow them to meet the Recommendations to Promote Social Distancing and Reduce Transmission.

2. Travel permitted for unsafe homes. Individuals whose residences are unsafe or become unsafe, such as victims of domestic violence, are permitted and urged to leave their home and stay at a safe alternative location.

D. Public transit. People riding on public transit must comply with the Recommendations to Promote Social Distancing and Reduce Transmission as defined in Subsection 2(A) to the greatest extent feasible.

Section 3. Orders for Businesses and Parks.

For the reasons and pursuant to the authority set forth above, the undersigned orders as follows:

A. Most Businesses and Organizations Can Be Open. All businesses that are not closed under Section 5 may operate. Some businesses must operate under restrictions, as stated in Sections 3, 4, 6, and 7 of this Executive Order.

B. Requirements Specific to Retail Businesses.

Retail Businesses that operate during the effective period of this Executive Order must:

l. Limit customer occupancy to not more than 50% of stated fire capacity. Retail Businesses that do not have a stated fire capacity must limit customer occupancy to twelve (12) customers for every one thousand (1000) square feet of the location's total square footage, including the parts of the location that are not accessible to customers.

1. Limit customer occupancy so that customers can stay six (6) feet apart, even if this requires reducing occupancy beneath the 50% limit stated above.

2. Direct customers to stay at least six (6) feet apart from one another and from workers, except at point of sale if applicable.

3. Mark six (6) feet of spacing in lines at point of sale and in other high-traffic areas for customers, such as at deli counters and near high-volume products.

4. Perform frequent and routine environmental cleaning and disinfection of high-touch areas with an EPA-approved disinfectant for SARS-CoV-2 (the virus that causes COVID- 19).

5. Provide, whenever available, hand sanitizer (at least 60% alcohol); systematically and frequently check and refill hand sanitizer stations; and provide soap and hand drying materials at sinks.

6. Conduct daily symptom screening of workers, using a standard interview questionnaire of symptoms, before workers enter the workplace.

7. Immediately send symptomatic workers home.

8. Have a plan in place for immediately isolating workers from the workplace if symptoms develop.

9. Post signage at the main entrances that reminds people to stay six (6) feet apart for social distancing, requests people who are or who have recently been symptomatic not to enter, and notifies customers of the Retail Business's reduced capacity.

The North Carolina Department of Health and Human Services ("NCDHHS") will make available on its website a sample screening checklist questionnaire and sample signs that may be used to meet the requirements above. Retail Businesses do not need to use the NCDHHS sample questionnaires and signs to meet the requirements of this Executive Order.

C. Additional Recommendations Specific to Retail Businesses.

Retail Businesses that operate during the effective period of this Executive Order are strongly encouraged to do the following:

Direct workers to stay at least six (6) feet apart from one another and from customers, to the greatest extent possible.

1. Provide designated times for seniors and other high-risk populations to access services.

2. Develop and use systems that allow for online, email, or telephone ordering, no-contact curbside or drive-through pickup or home delivery, and contact-free checkout.

3. High-volume Retail Businesses, such as grocery stores and pharmacies, are strongly encouraged to take the following additional measures to reduce transmission:

a. Use acrylic or plastic shields at cash registers.

b. Clearly mark designated entry and exit points.

c. Provide assistance with routing through aisles in the store.

4. Take all the additional actions listed in Subsection 3(D) below.

D. Recommendations for All Businesses (Retail or Other).

All businesses that operate during the effective period of this Executive Order are strongly encouraged to:

1. Continue to promote telework and limit non-essential travel whenever possible.

2. Promote social distancing by reducing the number of people coming to the office, by providing six (6) feet of distance between desks, and/or by staggering shifts.

3. Limit face-to-face meetings to no more than ten (1 0) workers.

4. Promote hygiene, including frequent hand-washing and use of hand sanitizer.

5. Recommend workers wear cloth Face Coverings; provide workers with Face Coverings; and provide information on proper use, removal, and washing of cloth Face Coverings. A Face Covering functions to protect other people more than the wearer.

6. Make accommodations for workers who are at high risk of severe illness from COVID-19, for example, by having high-risk workers work in positions that are not public-facing or by allowing teleworking where possible.

7. Encourage sick workers to stay home and provide support to do so with a sick leave policy.

8. Follow the CDC guidance if a worker has been diagnosed with COVID- 19.

9. Provide workers with education about COVID-19 prevention strategies, using methods like videos, webinars, or FAQs.

10. Promote information on help lines for workers such as 21 1 and the Hope4NC Helpline.

E. Parks and Trails.

1. All people in North Carolina are encouraged to engage in outdoor activities, so long as they do not form prohibited Mass Gatherings and are engaged in Allowable Activities under this Executive Order. State parks and trails may reopen upon the general Effective Date of this Executive Order. However, because public playground equipment may increase spread of COVID-19, public playgrounds remain closed during the effective phase of this Executive Order, including public playground equipment located in parks.

2. Park operators shall follow the requirements for Retail Businesses listed in Subsection (B) above, and they are strongly encouraged to follow the recommendations for Retail Businesses and the recommendations for all businesses in Subsections (C) and (D) above.

Section 4. Orders for Restricted Business Types.

For the reasons and pursuant to the authority set forth above, the undersigned orders as follows:

A. Restaurants.

1. Restaurants may remain open if consumption occurs off-premises. Restaurants may do business only to the extent that consumption of food and beverages occurs off-premises through such means as in-house delivery, third-party delivery, drive-through, curbside pick-up, and carry-out. Schools and other entities that provide free food services to students or members of the public may continue to do so under this Executive Order when the food is provided for carry-out, drive-through, or delivery.

2. Restaurants should follow social distancing and transmission reduction recommendations. Restaurants are encouraged to comply with the Recommendations to Promote Social Distancing and Reduce Transmission, including use of Face Coverings, when providing

carry-out, drive-through, and delivery services. These coverings function to protect other people, more than the wearer.

3. Further orders. The Governor, in consultation with and at the recommendation of the Secretary of Health and Human Services, the State Emergency Management Director, and the State Health Director, orders the following limitations on the sale of food and beverages to carry-out, drive-through, and delivery only:

a. The Secretary of Health and Human Services, pursuant to N.C. Gen. Stat.

130A-20(a), has determined that the seating areas of restaurants and bars constitute an imminent hazard for the spread of COVID-19 and that, to abate the imminent hazard, restaurants must be restricted to carry-out, drive-through, and delivery only and bars must close, and has issued an order of abatement dated May 4, 2020.

b. The undersigned directs that restaurants are restricted to carry-out, drive-through, and delivery only.

4. No sit-down service. Sit-down food or beverage service is prohibited at any kind of businesses, including but not limited to grocery stores, pharmacies, convenience stores, gas stations and charitable food distribution sites.

B. Bars.

1. Bars are directed to not serve alcoholic beverages for onsite consumption.

2. This Executive Order does not direct the closure of retail beverage venues that provide for the sale of beer, wine, and liquor for off-site consumption only. It also does not require the closure of production operations at breweries, wineries, or distilleries.

3. If the Alcoholic Beverage Control Commission (the "ABC Commission") identifies other state laws, regulations, and policies that may affect bars, restaurants, and other dining establishments identified in Subsections 4(A)-(B) of this Executive Order, it is directed to inform the Office of the Governor in writing. Upon written authorization from the Office of the Governor, the ABC Commission may interpret flexibly, modify, or waive those state laws, regulations and policies, as appropriate, and to the maximum extent permitted under applicable state and federal law, to effectuate the purposes of this Executive Order.

C. Child Care.

1. Must operate in compliance with NCDHHS guidelines. Child care facilities may be open only if they operate in full compliance with Executive Order No. 130 and all guidelines issued by NCDHHS.

2. Expanding children that may be served. The relevant language in Subsection 2(C) of Executive Order No. 130 is amended and replaced by the following:

Children that may be served. **Child Care Facilities** approved by NCDHHS to operate under the Emergency Facility Guidelines shall provide child care only to the following persons:

1. Children of anyone who performs work on behalf of a business or operation that is not closed by an Executive Order; or

2. Children of anyone who is leaving the home to seek employment; or

3. Children who are receiving child welfare services; or

4. Children who are homeless or who are living in unstable or unsafe living arrangements.

3. Term. Section 2 of Executive Order No. 130 shall remain in effect through 5:00 pm on May 22, 2020.

D. Day Camps and Programs for Children and Teens.

1. Must operate in compliance with NCDHHS guidelines. Day camps and programs may operate only if they are in full compliance with the Interim Coronavirus Disease 2019 (COVID-19) Guidance for Day Camp or Program Settings Serving Children and Teens. Day programs and camps for adults are not covered by this section.

2. No sports or other activities without social distancing. Day camps and programs may not allow sports except for sports where close contact is not required, and day camps may not allow activities where campers would not maintain at least six (6) feet social distancing from one another.

3. Day camps within another business or operation. Day camps and programs operating within a business, facility, or location closed by Subsection 5(B) of this Executive Order or at a school may open for the purpose of the day camp or program, but must otherwise remain closed to the general public. To the extent day camps permit swimming by camp attendees, local health departments may permit the pool's usage for attendees of the day camp, but not for the general public.

4. No overnight camps. Overnight camps and programs for children or adults may not operate.

E. Schools.

1. School facilities remain closed for in-person instruction. Consistent with Executive Orders No. 1 17 and 120, public school facilities are to remain closed as in-person instructional settings for students for the remainder of the 2019-2020 school year.

2. School and health officials to continue efforts. NCDHHS, the North Carolina Department of Public Instruction ("NCDPI"), and the North Carolina State Board of Education are directed to continue to work together to maintain and implement measures to provide for the

health, nutrition, safety, educational needs, and well-being of children during the school closure period.

3. Graduation and other year-end ceremonies. Local school boards and superintendents will determine whether to conduct graduation and/or other year-end ceremonies. If local school leaders elect to hold graduation ceremonies or similar events, then those gatherings must operate in compliance with Executive Orders and NCDPI/NCDHHS guidelines in effect at the time of the cvent. Local school leaders are encouraged to engage with students and families to identify the best solutions for their communities. Local plans should include consultation with local public health officials and, where appropriate, local law enforcement.

Section 5. Orders for Businesses to Remain Closed.

A. Personal Care and Grooming Businesses.

1. The ability to practice the social distancing necessary to reasonably protect against COVID-19 is significantly reduced in certain establishments where individuals are in extended close proximity or where service personnel are in direct contact with clients. Therefore, personal care and grooming businesses, including but not limited to the following, are ordered to close:

>Barber Shops
>
>Beauty Salons (including but not limited to waxing and hair removal centers)
>
>Hair Salons
>
>Nail Salons/Manicure/Pedicure Providers
>
>Tattoo Parlors
>
>Tanning Salons

 Massage Therapists (except that massage therapists may provide medical massage therapy services upon the specific referral of a medical or naturopathic healthcare provider).

B. Entertainment Facilities without a Retail or Dining Component.

l. In addition to the restrictions on Mass Gatherings identified in Section 6 of this Executive Order, entertainment facilities that operate within a confined indoor or outdoor space and do not offer a retail or dining component are ordered to close. Any retail or dining component within an entertainment facility may operate solely for retail or dining, but those components must comply with the restrictions set out in Subsection 4(A) of this Executive Order.

2. Entertainment facilities restricted by this Subsection include, but are not limited to, the following types of business:

Bingo Parlors, including bingo sites operated by charitable organizations

Bowling Alleys

Indoor Exercise Facilities (e.g., gyms, yoga studios, martial arts facilities, indoor trampoline and rock-climbing facilities, Health Clubs, Fitness Centers, and Gyms

Indoor/Outdoor Pools

Live Performance Venues

Movie Theaters

Skating Rinks

Spas, including health spas

Gaming and business establishments which allow gaming activities (e.g., video poker, gaming, sweepstakes, video games, arcade games, pinball machines or other computer, electronic or mechanical devices played for amusement).

Section 6. Mass Gatherings Prohibited.

Prohibition. Mass Gatherings are prohibited. "Mass Gathering" means an event or convening that brings together more than ten (10) persons at the same time in a single space, such as an auditorium, stadium, arena, conference room, meeting hall, or any other confined indoor or outdoor space. This includes parades, fairs, and festivals.

Mass Gatherings do not include gatherings for health and safety, to look for and obtain goods and services, for work, for worship, or exercise of First Amendment rights, or for receiving governmental services. A Mass Gathering does not include normal operations at airports, bus and train stations or stops, medical facilities, shopping malls, and shopping centers. However, in these settings, people must follow the Recommendations to Promote Social Distancing and Reduce Transmission as much as possible, and they should circulate within the space so that there is no sustained contact between people.

B. Dividing one event or convening into multiple sessions. Nothing in this Executive Order prohibits holding several events or convenings instead of one so that at any time, no more than ten (10) people are gathered in the same space. Organizations that need to hold events or convenings in a single space are encouraged to hold multiple sessions so that no more than ten (10) people are present at a time. In addition, nothing in this Executive Order prohibits holding meetings remotely, and all people in North Carolina are encouraged to hold gatherings electronically so that large groups can meet.

C. Outdoor meetings if possible. Because the risk of COVID-19 spread is much greater in an indoor setting, any gatherings of more than ten (10) people that are allowed under Subsection 6(A) shall take place outdoors unless impossible.

D. Funerals. Notwithstanding the above, and in an effort to promote human dignity and limit suffering, Mass Gatherings at funerals are permitted for up to fifty (50) people. People meeting at a funeral should observe the Recommendations to Promote Social Distancing and Reduce Transmission to the extent practicable.

E. Drive-ins. Events are not prohibited Mass Gatherings if the participants all stay within their cars, such as at a drive-in movie theater.

F.   Households. A household where more than ten (10) people reside is not a Mass Gathering.

Section 7.   Long Term Care.

For the reasons and pursuant to the authority set forth above, the undersigned orders as follows:

A. Long Term Care Visitation Limitations.

1. Long term care facilities shall restrict visitation of all visitors and non-essential health care personnel, except for certain compassionate care situations, for example, an end-of-life situation.

2. This restriction does not include essential health care personnel.

3. For purposes of this Subsection 7(A) only, long term care facilities include all of the following:

a. Skilled nursing facilities;

b. Adult care homes;

c. Family care homes;

d. Mental health group homes; and

e. Intermediate care facilities for individuals with intellectual disabilities.

B. Long Term Care Risk Mitigation Measures.

1. Scope of this Subsection. This Subsection of this Executive Order places mandatory requirements on skilled nursing facilities. This Subsection strongly encourages the same measures, to the extent possible given constraints on the availability of personal protective equipment, for other kinds of long-term care facilities, including adult care homes, family care homes, mental health group homes, and intermediate care facilities for individuals with intellectual disabilities.

2. Mitigation measures. Skilled nursing facilities shall:

a. Remind workers to stay home when they are ill and prevent any workers who are ill from coming to work and/or staying at work.

b. Screen all workers at the beginning of their shift for fever and respiratory symptoms. This shall include:

261

i. Actively taking that worker's temperature.

ii. Documenting an absence of any shortness of breath, any new cough or changes in cough, and any sore throat. If the worker is ill, the facility must have the worker put on a facemask and leave the workplace.

iii. Canceling communal dining and all group activities, including internal and external activities.

iv. Implementing universal use of a facemask for all workers while in the facility, assuming supplies are available.

v. Actively monitor all residents upon admission, and at least daily, for fever and respiratory symptoms (shortness of breath, new cough or change in cough, and sore throat), and shall continue to monitor residents.

vi. Notify the local health department immediately about either of the following:

1. Any resident with new, confirmed, or suspected COVID-19.

2. A cluster of residents or workers with symptoms of respiratory illness. A "cluster" of residents or workers means three (3) or more people (residents or workers) with new-onset respiratory symptoms in a period of 72 hours.

C. Other kinds of long-term care facilities. Adult care homes, family care homes, mental health group homes, and intermediate care facilities for individuals with intellectual disabilities are strongly encouraged to follow the mitigation measures listed in Subsections 7(B)(2)(b)(i) through (vi) above, assuming supplies are available.

Effective Date and Duration. This Section of this Executive Order shall remain in effect unless repealed, replaced, or rescinded by another applicable Executive Order.

Section 8. Local Orders.

For the reasons and pursuant to the authority set forth above, the undersigned orders as follows:

A. Effect on local emergency management orders.

1. Most of the restrictions in this Executive Order are minimum requirements. and local governments can impose greater restrictions. The undersigned recognizes that the impact of COVID-19 has been and will likely continue to be different in different parts of North Carolina. Urban areas have seen more rapid and significant spread than most rural areas of the state. As such, the undersigned acknowledges that counties and cities may deem it necessary to adopt ordinances and issue state of emergency declarations which impose restrictions or prohibitions to the extent authorized under North Carolina law, such as on the activity of people and businesses, to a greater degree than in this Executive Order. To that end, nothing herein, except where specifically stated below in Subsections A(2) and A(3) of this Section, is intended to limit or prohibit counties and cities in North Carolina from

enacting ordinances and issuing state of emergency declarations which impose greater restrictions or prohibitions to the extent authorized under North Carolina law.

2. Local restrictions cannot restrict state or federal government operations. Notwithstanding Subsection 8(A)(1) above, no county or city ordinance or declaration shall have the effect of restricting or prohibiting governmental operations of the State or the United States.

3. Local restrictions cannot set different retail requirements. Notwithstanding Subsection 8(A) (1) above, in an effort to create uniformity across the state for Retail Businesses that may continue to operate, the undersigned amends all local prohibitions and restrictions imposed under any local state of emergency declarations to remove any language that sets a different maximum occupancy standard for Retail Businesses or otherwise directly conflicts with Subsections 3(B)(1)—(2) of this Executive Order. The undersigned also hereby prohibits during the pendency of this Executive Order the adoption of any prohibitions and restrictions under any local state of emergency declarations that set a different maximum occupancy standard for Retail Businesses or otherwise directly conflict with Subsections 3(B) (l)-(2) of this Executive Order.

B. Mandatory local government operations.

1. To the extent that local government functions are required under state and federal law, the undersigned directs the appropriate local government agencies and officials to continue to exercise their responsibilities, including but not limited to local county Department of Social Services ("DSS") offices, Health Departments, Registers of Deeds, and other local government functions that are required to protect lives and property.

2. Notwithstanding Subsection 8(B)(1) above, local governments are strongly encouraged to follow the Requirements Specific to Retail Businesses in Subsection 3(B) and Recommendations for Retail Businesses in Subsection 3(C) for functions where members of the public enter a space to receive or use government services. Local governments are also strongly encouraged to follow the Recommendations for All Businesses (Retail or Other) included in Subsection 3(D).

Section 9. Extension of Price Gouging Period.

For the reasons and pursuant to the authority set forth above, the undersigned orders as follows:

Pursuant to N.C. Gen. Stat. 166A-19.23, the undersigned extends the prohibition against excessive pricing, as provided in N.C. Gen. Stat. 75-37 and 75-38, from the issuance of Executive Order No. 116 through 5:00 pm on May 22, 2020.

The undersigned further hereby encourages the North Carolina Attorney General to use all resources available to monitor reports of abusive trade practices towards consumers and make readily available opportunities to report to the public any price gouging and unfair or deceptive trade practices under Chapter 75 of the North Carolina General Statutes.

Section 10. No Private Right of Action.

This Executive Order is not intended to create, and does not create, any individual right, privilege, or benefit, whether substantive or procedural, enforceable at law or in equity by any party against the State of North Carolina, its agencies, departments, political subdivisions, or other entities, or any officers, employees, or agents thereof, or any emergency management worker (as defined in N.C. Gen. Stat. 166A-19.60) or any other person.

Section 11. Savings Clause.

If any provision of this Executive Order or its application to any person or circumstances is held invalid by any court of competent jurisdiction, this invalidity does not affect any other provision or application of this Executive Order, which can be given effect without the invalid provision or application. To achieve this purpose, the provisions of this Executive Order are declared to be severable.

Section 12. Distribution.

I hereby order that this Executive Order be: (1) distributed to the news media and other organizations calculated to bring its contents to the attention of the general public; (2) promptly filed with the Secretary of the North Carolina Department of Public Safety, the Secretary of State, and the superior court clerks in the counties to which it applies, unless the circumstances of the State of Emergency would prevent or impede such filing; and (3) distributed to others as necessary to ensure proper implementation of this Executive Order.

Section 13. Enforcement

A.   Pursuant to N.C. Gen. Stat. 166A-19.30(a)(2), the provisions of this Executive Order shall be enforced by state and local law enforcement officers.

B. A violation of this Executive Order may be subject to prosecution pursuant to N.C. Gen. Stat. ss 166A-19.30(d), and is punishable as a Class 2 misdemeanor in accordance with N.C. Gen. Stat. 14-288.20A.

C. Nothing in this Executive Order shall be construed to preempt or overrule a court order regarding an individual's conduct (e.g., a Domestic Violence Protection Order or similar orders limiting an individual's access to a particular place).

Section 14. Effective Date

This Executive Order is effective at 5:00 pm on May 8, 2020.

Section 7 of this Executive Order shall remain in effect for the period stated in Subsection 7(C) of this Executive Order. The remainder of this **Order shall remain in effect through 5:00 pm on May 22, 2020** unless repealed, replaced, or rescinded by another applicable Executive Order. An Executive Order rescinding the Declaration of the State of Emergency will automatically rescind this Executive Order.

IN WITNESS WHEREOF, 1 have hereunto signed my name and affixed the Great Seal of the State of North Carolina at the Capitol in the City of Raleigh, this 5th day of May in the year of our Lord two thousand and twenty.

Roy Cooper, Governor

May 8, 2020 Statistics

Globally: 3,907,055 cases with 272,578 deaths.

United States: 1,271,775 cases with 76,368 deaths.

North Carolina statistics on May 8, 2020:[89]

Cases	TESTED	Deaths	Counties
13,868 527	178,613	527	99

Currently 515 hospitalized in North Carolina.

Age groups:

0-17	3 % of cases and 0 % deaths.
18-24	7 % of cases and 0 % of deaths.
25-49	42 % of cases and 3 % of deaths.
50-64	26 % of cases and 11 % of deaths.
65+	22 % of cases and 86 % of deaths.

By Race/Ethnicity on May 8, 2020:[90]

Laboratory-Confirmed Cases   % Laboratory-Confirmed Cases

Deaths from COVID-19   % Deaths from COVID-19

Total with known race	1	10,316	500

---

[89]   https://www.ncdhhs.gov/divisions/public-health/COVID19/COVID-19-nc-case-count#by-race-ethnicity.
May 8, 2020
[90] https://www.ncdhhs.gov/divisions/public-health/COVID19/COVID-19-nc-case-count#by-race-ethnicity.
May 8, 2020.

	Cases	Cases	Deaths	Deaths
American Indian Alaskan Native	101	1%	1	0%
Asian	254	2%	6	1%
Black or African American	3,679	36%	172	34%
Native Hawaiian / Pacific Islander	22	0%	1	0%
White	5,430	53%	302	60%
Other	830	8%	18	4%
Total with known ethnicity	2	9,227		447
Hispanic	2,195	24%	18	4%
Non-Hispanic	7,032	76%	429	96%

1 Race data are missing for 3,552 laboratory-confirmed cases and 27 deaths.

2 Ethnicity data are missing for 4,641 laboratory-confirmed cases and 80 deaths.

All data are preliminary and may change as cases are investigated.

NC Cases by Gender on May 8, 2020:

48% are male   50% are female   2% are Unknown

NC Deaths by Gender on May 8, 2020:

54% of deaths were male.

46% of deaths were female.

2% of deaths were unknown gender.

The latest modeling on May 8, 2020 indicates that in North Carolina:

Recent trends indicate that the viral spread has slowed down a bit in North Carolina. Most of the localized outbreaks in North Carolina occurred in congregate work and residential settings. Hospital care is sufficient at this timeCOVID-19 reported cases continue to rise. Officials say that the rise could be attributed to the rise in the number of cases tested.

In Brunswick County the county departments request that individuals email or call first to get an appointment for an in-person visit if needed. Social distancing is still recommended and folks are still encouraged to stay home, although some businesses are beginning to open for business. Restaurants remain closed with take- out service or delivery.

Congress has approved 1.57 billion in Federal Aid for PPE, testing, contract tracing, small business loans, and food banks. The end of grade testing and has set the school start date as August 17th of this year.

Phase One is getting implemented but social distancing is still highly recommended. Retail businesses will be opening at 50% capacity under conditions previously noted in the Governor Cooper North Carolina State mandates.

On the horizon, more cases are expected. Social distancing measure are being reviewed for effectiveness with modifications as needed. Surge capacity at hospitals and medical facilities are requesting more clinicians and PPE. COVID-19 testing at the point of care will be offered and rapid results available in less than an hour are going to be coming. Trials are ongoing for antiviral therapy.

North Carolina Counties on May 8, 2020:[91]

County	Laboratory-Confirmed Cases	Deaths
Alamance County	149	3
Alexander County	8	0
Alleghany County	7	0
Anson County	37	0
Ashe County	7	0
Beaufort County	24	0
Bertie County	58	2
Bladen County	50	1
Brunswick County	49	2

---

[91] https://www.ncdhhs.gov/divisions/public-health/COVID19/COVID-19-nc-case-count#by-counties-map. May 8, 2020.

Buncombe County	88	4
Burke County	128	11
Cabarrus County	338	17
Caldwell County	52	0
Camden County	2	0
Carteret County	29	3
Caswell County	38	1
Catawba County	67	1
Chatham County	435	11
Cherokee County	18	1
Chowan County	8	0
Clay County	5	0
Cleveland County	50	2
Columbus County	186	13
Craven County	49	4
Cumberland County	342	9
Currituck County	9	0
Dare County	14	1
Davidson County	199	10
Davie County	31	2
Duplin County	180	3
Durham County	829	31
Edgecombe County	139	7
Forsyth County	353	5
Franklin County	111	20
Gaston County	161	4
Gates County	10	0
Graham County	2	0

Granville County	159	5
Greene County	34	0
Guilford County	553	38
Halifax County	82	1
Harnett County	207	12
Haywood County	16	0
Henderson County	218	24
Hertford County	46	1
Hoke County	117	0
Hyde County	1	0
Iredell County	141	5
Jackson County	21	1
Johnston County	191	16
Jones County	18	2
Lee County	238	1
Lenoir County	105	4
Lincoln County	39	0
Macon County	3	1
Madison County	1	0
Martin County	28	1
McDowell County	29	1
Mecklenburg County	1,989	58
Mitchell County	5	0
Montgomery County	41	2
Moore County	109	9
Nash County	116	3
New Hanover County	95	3
Northampton County	102	7

Onslow County	53	2
Orange County	244	32
Pamlico County	8	0
Pasquotank County	75	3
Pender County	23	1
Perquimans County	14	2
Person County	29	1
Pitt County	160	2
Polk County	31	0
Randolph County	307	5
Richmond County	81	2
Robeson County	327	4
Rockingham County	38	2
Rowan County	467	24
Rutherford County	149	5
Sampson County	136	1
Scotland County	36	0
Stanly County	29	4
Stokes County	11	0
Surry County	30	1
Swain County	5	0
Transylvania County	7	0
Tyrrell County	4	0
Union County	284	15
Vance County	153	11
Wake County	986	22
Warren County	22	0
Washington County	25	3

Watauga County	9	0
Wayne County	715	12
Wilkes County	198	1
Wilson County	199	8
Yadkin County	39	1
Yancey County	7	0

Brunswick County Residents: 49 cases with 2 deaths. May 8, 2020.

Number of Test Samples reported to the County: 1015

Pending Test Sample Results: 42

Positive Tests Results reported to county: 49

Negative Test Results reported to county: 1,604

Brunswick County Non-residents: 10 known cases. May 8, 2020.

0 isolated at home.

0 isolated at hospital.

2 deaths.

4 currently recovered.

3 transferred monitoring to home residence.

70 % male and 30% female died.

40% ages 25-49 death rate.

10% ages 50-64 death rate, and

50% over the age of 65 death rate.

Statistics, statistics, statistics…the numbers can almost become a complicated puzzle as one reads through this text. While it is important to have access to the latest numbers, it is *history* to report than from the beginning so that one can readily see how the numbers have increased in such a short period of time. While they will continue increasing, for the purpose of this book, statistical numbers will be finalized in 2021.

No doubt the numbers will increase, and this author encourages the ready to pencil in additional information in the appropriate places where you have an interest. It is sad that the experts predict that the death rate has approached over 500,000 in the United States by March of 2021.

By **March 19, 2021,** Brunswick County found itself with the following statistics and in a decline of cases, hospitalizations and deaths; hoping the end of this pandemic was in sight. Time will tell.

COVID-19 Partner Briefing Operational Day 373 - March 19, 2021

Brunswick County Health and Human Services

Case Counts

122,079,358 cases globally (2,695,729 deaths)

29,708,451 in the United States (540,533 deaths)

*893,229 cases in North Carolina (11,805 deaths)

NCDHHS *8,433 cases in Brunswick County (141 deaths)

4% Daily Positive Test Results

970 currently hospitalized

1915 New Cases reported on this date

North Carolina   893,229 Known COVID-19 cases

970 Currently Hospitalized

11,805 Deaths

Patients Presumed to be Recovered 874,509

Gender	Percent of Cases	Percent of Deaths
Male	47%	52%
Female	53%	48%

Age Group	Percent of Cases	Percent of Deaths
0-17	12%	0%
18-24	14%	0%
25-49	39%	3%

50-64	20%	13%
65+	15%	83%

Brunswick County Residents

    8,433 Known COVID-19 cases

    285 Active cases

    141 Deaths

    8,007 Patients presumed to be recovered

Gender/Age	Cases	Deaths
Male	46%	56%
Female	54%	44%
Age 0 to 17	11%	0%
Age 18-24	9%	0%
Age 25-49	31%	7%
Age 50-64	23%	6%
Age 65+	27%	87%

March 19, 2021: Current studies show that as many as 10% to 50% of COVID-19 cases may initially report to be asymptomatic.

After going upwards to almost 900 active cases a day, Brunswick County is now down to just less than 300 active cases. If this trend continues, we truly will be getting to the other side of COVID, at least for now.

As of April 26, 2021: Case Counts

    147,350,284 cases globally (3,112,311 deaths)

    32,092,128 in the United States (572,287 deaths)

    *962,623 cases in North Carolina (12,560 deaths)

    NCDHHS *9,006 cases in Brunswick County (150 deaths)

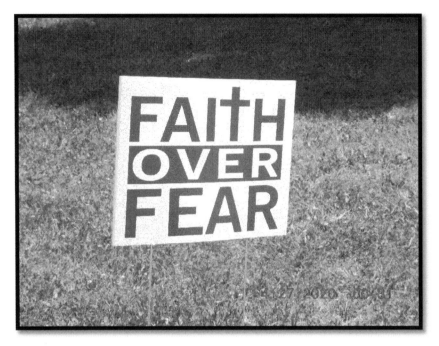

Figure 69 Yard Sign.

284

Made in the USA
Columbia, SC
20 June 2021

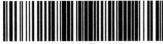